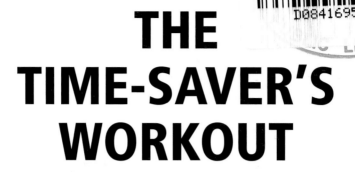

THE TIME-SAVER'S WORKOUT

A Revolutionary New Fitness Plan that Dispels Myths and Optimizes Results

JOHN LITTLE

Author of
Bruce Lee: The Art of Expressing the Human Body and *Max Contraction Training,*
Co-author of *Body By Science*

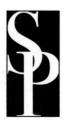

Skyhorse Publishing

Skyhorse Publishing books may be purchased in bulk at special discounts for sales promotion, corporate gifts, fund-raising, or educational purposes. Special editions can also be created to specifications. For details, contact the Special Sales Department, Skyhorse Publishing, 307 West 36th Street, 11th Floor, New York, NY 10018 or info@skyhorsepublishing.com.

Skyhorse® and Skyhorse Publishing® are registered trademarks of Skyhorse Publishing, Inc.®, a Delaware corporation.

Visit our website at www.skyhorsepublishing.com.

10 9 8 7 6 5 4 3 2 1

Library of Congress Cataloging-in-Publication Data is available on file.

Cover design by Tom Lau
Cover photo credit: iStock

ISBN: 978-1-5107-3330-5
Ebook ISBN: 978-1-5107-3331-2

Printed in China

This book is designed to provide accurate and authoritative information with respect to the subject matter covered. While every attempt is made to provide accurate information, the author or publisher cannot be held accountable for errors or omissions. Be sure to consult a physician before beginning any exercise routine.

To my wife, Terri,
and our children Riley, Taylor, Brandon, and Ben

TABLE OF CONTENTS

PART THREE: EXERCISE—A NEW PARADIGM

"Do not labor uselessly at what helps not at all."
—Aeschylus

INTRODUCTION

The most precious commodity in our lives is time. Once spent it is irretrievable, impossible to get back. Each of our lives is made up of a finite amount of time that invariably ends. Some people have the luxury of having lots of what is called "spare time" and are consumed with looking for ways to fill it, but most of us are hard-pressed to do what we need to do within the modest allotment of time that we have. Our lives are more complicated these days; some of us work more than two jobs, and some of us have children who require what little time we have away from work.

Exercise is considered to be important to many of us for the purpose of staying healthy enough and capable enough to carry on with what we need to do in our lives. But are we doing enough of it? Should we be making sacrifices in other areas of our lives in order to free up more valuable time in order to ensure that we are doing everything that we should in order to stay fit and healthy—even if we only have time to apply these health and fitness rewards to our work and in tending to our relationship commitments? Would it surprise you to learn that this author believes that we're already spending way too much time exercising, and that we could free up most of the time that we are devoting to exercise right now and probably be fitter, healthier, and a hell of a lot happier as a result? I don't believe exercise should be the reason for your life, but rather an adjunct to it. Moreover, I don't believe the evidence supports the need for exercise classes, multiple-day-per-week visits to the gym, or taking out a second mortgage on your home to purchase nutritional supplements. If you've been kind of thinking along these same lines yourself, then welcome to the minimalist approach—a movement toward trimming away the unessential things in your life to free up more of that all-too-rare commodity of time.

Those people who presently believe that they require hours and hours of exercise each week in order to be fully functional and healthy have, in my humble opinion, been played for suckers by the commercial interests that have dominated the exercise (and "health") industry ever since its inception. You may count yourself among them; perhaps you've already purchased the $100 yoga pants, the $150 pair of running shoes, the cowhide weightlifting gloves, and the cupboard full of vitamin and herbal supplements. But don't feel bad, as you're not alone; most of us have been taken in by fitness hucksterism in one form or another over the years.

In 1887 the philosopher Friedrich Nietzsche released a short philosophical novel entitled *Thus Spake Zarathustra*. It was a powerful little book containing many powerful statements, but one statement in particular has proven to be prophetically true over the past century:

> Where the marketplace begins, there begins also the noise of the great actors, and the buzzing of the poison-flies.

And while Europe's great iconoclast never envisioned the goings on within the fitness industry when he penned these words, I'm certain that he would have agreed that the sentiment most readily applies. Indeed, the "great actors" have descended upon the fitness world in the form of celebrities and self-appointed exercise and nutrition gurus, with the result that the exercise marketplace now seems to be constantly abuzz with "poison-flies"; i.e., carriers of erroneous information, with the perhaps not entirely unpredictable result that a contagion has spread in the form of harmful falsehoods.

Every new approach in exercise is brought before the public as being the "ultimate" and each has its adherents that certainly look the part. But if you pull far enough back from the din of the marketplace a pattern begins to emerge and that is that the "ultimate truth" in the health and fitness industry changes before us in kaleidoscopic fashion; one week dietary fat intake is the sole reason our society is obese; the next week it's the fault of carbohydrates; another week aerobics (steppers, elipiticals, treadmills, running) is the best type of exercise one could perform for his or her health, and the next week it's yoga. The Internet has only compounded this problem of contradictory information, as almost everyone who posts their views online does so with an air of authority and is quick to decry those methods that differ from their own. The silent majority who earnestly seek simple and truthful answers to their most basic of health and fitness questions are left confused, as the answers they are presented with are anything but simple and seldom truthful.

Then there is the transitory societal standard of how a male and female body should appear, which seems to shift and change with each passing decade like clouds in the sky. As hard as it may be for our youth of today to imagine, it wasn't always *de rigueur* to be thin with highly defined muscles. As proof one need only to look to our celebrities from the past. Actors from the 1950s, such as Marlon Brando and Marilyn Monroe, both of whom influenced millions with their physical appearance and were looked upon as representing the ideals of their day in terms of male and female body types, are, by present-day standards, considered to be rather pedestrian in terms of their respective appearances. Even further back, the overflowing ladies of Rubens, the buxom lasses of Rembrandt, and even Raphael's Madonnas were all rather physically prosperous. Alas, no more. Today our actors have bodies that look like competitive bodybuilders (and many of them are willing to take the steroids and other drugs necessary to achieve that look), while the models who pose for the cameras of corporations such as Victoria Secret and Calvin Klein likewise display a professional bodybuilder's low level of body fat and are held up as representing the standard of how we should look in our undergarments. Our film stars, models, and elite athletes have both created and continued to fuel a mythology of image that not only has altered our perception of how we think we should look, but that has also spawned a national (indeed, a global) desire to become slimmer and leaner. And the primary (if not sole) beneficiary of all of this attention to muscles and leanness has been the health and fitness industry.

Walk into any health food store or thumb through the pages of any fitness magazine and there on the shelves and pages are products proclaiming transformative (and in many cases spectacularly transformative) properties that can be yours upon purchase. A myriad fitness centers join in the call, beckoning us with the allure of dramatic improvements in our appearance being but the purchase of a gym membership away. A casual stroll through any of these facilities reveals a smorgasbord of programs and high-tech machinery that, we are assured, in themselves, yield the potential to completely transform our bodies and take us from how we look right now to how we want to look. On display are various cardio machines to improve our aerobic health, yoga classes to increase our limberness and flexibility, and barbells and resistance training machines to build up our muscles and make us stronger.

If the whole "gym scene" doesn't hold appeal, you are told that you needn't worry—you can still obtain the fantastic results that you desire while training in the comfort of your own home. Many of us have evidently been seduced by this belief, as sales of home exercise equipment, particularly treadmills and resistance training devices such as BowFlex™ machines, have never been higher. Surprisingly, however, given such an abundance of services, information, and products that are currently available to make us slimmer, more energetic, and more attractive, one statistic has emerged that is rather puzzling—overall we're fatter, weaker, and less healthy now than at any other point in our species' history.[1] The question logically follows the statistic: with so many things that are now available for us to take and do to become healthier, stronger, leaner, and more energetic, why aren't we seeing an increase in the number of people becoming any more of any one of these things? In fact, quite the opposite would appear to be the case; i.e., that most of us are getting fatter, have less energy, and are in poorer health now than we were five years ago. How can this be? This book is an attempt to answer these questions and to suggest a means by which we can build (or at the very least preserve) our health and strength and change our appearances for the better without spending thousands of dollars in the health food store or the bulk of our lives in the gym.

THE EMPEROR'S NEW CLOTHES

Like most people who earned their living outside of the fitness industry, I once took as Gospel everything that was printed in the various fitness magazines. The articles were, presumably, written by leading experts and authorities in the field and, by comparison, who was I to question the insights of such highly esteemed authors? But then a terrible thing happened: I was granted entry into the inner sanctum of the industry when I accepted a job offer to write for one of the nation's top bodybuilding and fitness magazines. This publication (along with several other magazines it released under its masthead) had almost single-handedly shaped the fitness industry that we know today.

I wasn't at my new job long when it became clear that science, research, and dispensing truth were not particularly welcome guests in a domain where product sales and marketing held sway. Indeed, the only time "science" was brought into an article was when it could be extrapolated to support certain ingredients in a particular supplement that the publisher or one of his advertisers was selling. During my tenure at this publication I saw many articles get into print that contained questionable information and most of them were not even written by the physique champion (in the case of bodybuilding) whose name appeared on the article's byline. It quickly became apparent that any information that I wished to discover regarding the actual facts of diet and exercise would have to be pursued outside of company hours on my own time.

After four years of working on a daily basis in the fitness industry I left the magazine and began an independent career as an author and fitness researcher, which has continued unabated now for over 23 years. My time at the publication wasn't entirely unfruitful, however, as apart from revealing the Emperor's New Clothes of it all, it also opened my eyes to the preponderance of steroids (and other growth drugs) used in the fitness industry. It also made clear to me why any attempt by a normal person to ape the training and diet programs of professional bodybuilders or fitness models would typically end in failure and frustration.

It must be pointed out that exercise is a *massive* industry. It has been reported that Americans currently spend in excess of 60 billion dollars per year on gym memberships, weight loss products, workout clothing, and exercise equipment.[2] And while it has taken me over 20 years of daily practical research, I can now say with confidence what actually works, and to what degree, and what doesn't work. Among the data presented in this book are the following facts:

- Exercise (whether strength training or cardio) can sometimes make certain individuals less healthy and fatter.

- The human body will adapt, and often quite quickly, to *any* exercise program, which will rapidly diminish any beneficial effect that the exercise program might have yielded. I have labeled this phenomenon the C.E.P. (Conservation of Energy Phenomenon), and it applies not only to exercise, but to all activities (mental and physical).

- Extreme endurance activities such as triathlons and double marathons, rather than helping to increase one's longevity, can increase an individual's risk for germ-cell cancers.

- Genetic endowment, which is something that is essentially immutable, is the ultimate determinate of athletic success, and yet fitness professionals (who charge top dollar to young athletes and their parents in order to sell them the dream of making it big in professional sports) largely ignore it.

- It's almost in our DNA to avoid the very type of physical activity that will do us the most good.

- Taking large doses of food supplements might actually shorten your life and put you at greater risk for disease.

- Running, despite its popularity, is a very high-risk activity and is particularly harmful for women.

- Stretching to become more flexible or to recover more quickly from injury has been found to do neither of these things.

- Exercising for hours each week for cardiovascular health is no longer necessary or desirable.

- Resistance training, once considered to be the weak sister of exercise, is the best form of exercise one can engage in.

The above points are not based on my mere opinion, but rather on an intensive examination of the scientific literature as it applies to human beings and exercise. Apart from the critical analysis indicated above, I also hope with this book to impart something of positive value to the reader in the form of two exercise protocols that have been engineered to dramatically increase the metabolic component of an exercise session, resulting in a far more thorough activation of one's muscle fibers and metabolic pathways for complete and total fitness. In addition, these two protocols have been designed with an eye toward reducing the forces that most people expose themselves to when exercising, as well as the wear and tear components that typically attend the performance of most forms of physical activity, thus making them a far safer alternative to conventional forms of exercise.

However, before proceeding, I should mention an important fact. In my career as a personal trainer I've had clients with a wide array of fitness goals. Some have expressed a desire to become stronger; others have wanted to build bigger, more shapely muscles; still others have wanted to become stronger *without* building bigger, more shapely muscles, but most have wanted to lose fat, to increase their energy or endurance, and simply wanted to look different than they presently do, and to feel better about themselves. To this end I've had medical doctors fly halfway around the world to meet with me to learn of my methods and even had high-profile individuals such as Peak Performance Coach Tony Robbins write a foreword to one of my books and also fly me to Fiji to implement my methods before the cameras of a major national television network. While this may sound impressive to some, I would be remiss if I did not state at the outset that not all of my clients achieve their personal transformation goals. The reason for that, I believe, is that their goals are not based on reality; i.e., they have been oversold on just what exercise can accomplish. Fathers who wish for their sons to gain 30 pounds of solid muscle over the course of a summer of lifting weights in order to play better in their given sport and women who want to lose 25 pounds of body fat over the course of a few weeks in order to look good in their bathing suits for a forthcoming trip will find no words of comfort or encouragement within these pages. What they will find instead is a reality check and a means to better become what they are, rather than what they might wish to be.

I'm certainly aware that truth can often be an unwelcome guest in one's life when it runs contrary to one's desires, but it can also be a light that leads us out of the darkened catacombs of an industry that has always placed commerce above reality. Whatever our genetic potential yields from exercise, however great or small that potential may be, it is important for each of us to understand that genetic limits exist with regard to what exercise can accomplish. One who understands this is in large measure protected in advance against the delusions and disillusionments propagated by the fitness industry. Hopefully the minimalist approach outlined within the pages of this book will save the reader from wasting the most valuable commodity that we possess—time. Time that otherwise would be irretrievably lost chasing fitness industry rainbows that only seem to recede further into the ether the closer one gets to touching them.

—John Little

ACKNOWLEDGMENTS

Very rarely is any book (and particularly one on exercise) the result of a sudden stroke of genius on behalf of its author. In the case of this title the author was fortunate to have lit his lamp from many different torches, the two brightest being Mike Mentzer and Doug McGuff, M.D., the latter being in the author's humble opinion the brightest mind in exercise science today. To this end the author is beholden to these gentlemen for sharing their bounteous knowledge with him and allowing him to work with them on various books in the past. While the presentation of the facts contained within this book may be new to the lay reader, the student of exercise science will recognize much of the material and understand that very little is new, save for arrangement. If there is anything truly original here it will probably be unintentional and most likely regrettable to the author in later years as new data comes into the physical sciences. In any event, the author has done what he could to bring some perspective to the bigger picture of what exercise can and cannot accomplish for the vast majority of human beings.

The author would like to thank the following personal trainers for taking the time to contribute to the illustrations that appear in this book. Their (or their clients') demonstrating these protocols is not meant to imply that they use or advocate my methods, as many of them have evolved their own approaches to resistance training that are different from the author's. That they would nevertheless lend their time and image to these illustrations is considered a gesture of kindness and goodwill on their part for which the author is very grateful.

The following trainers are among the best in the world at what they do and if the reader finds his or herself in their neighborhood, you would do well to book an appointment with any one of these individuals:

Doug McGuff (Ultimate Exercise): http://www.drmcguff.com; Bill DeSimone (Optimal Exercise): http://www.optimalexercisenj .com; Bo Railey (Exercise Inc.): http://exerciseinc.com; Jeremy Hymers (who has no web address because he actually works for a living—or so he tells me on a weekly basis); Blair Wilson (Medx Precision Fitness): https://medxpf.com.

PART ONE
THE PROBLEM WITH EXERCISE

CHAPTER ONE

COFFEE TALK

I vividly recall a conversation I had with former bodybuilding champion Mike Mentzer back in 1992. We were both living in California at the time and, as I recall, it was a beautiful morning; the sun was shining brightly through a cloudless sky and the warm temperature facilitated genial conversation as we sat down at one of his favorite coffee shops in Santa Monica. Mike had competed against some of the world's best athletes in ABC television's "The Superstars" competition and had even won a score of bodybuilding titles such as Mr. America and Mr. Universe before retiring rather abruptly from competitive bodybuilding following the controversial Mr. Olympia contest in 1980. I asked him if he missed bodybuilding competition. He took a sip from his coffee and shook his head in the negative.

"Not at all."

"Why's that?"

"It's not relevant anymore. There was a time when I never thought I could say such a thing—I was obsessed by being a bodybuilder; I was young, innocent, naïve, and even stupid to some degree. But time goes on, and we mature and learn things."

"And what things have you learned that would cause you to reevaluate the number of hours you had devoted to building your body?" I queried.

"Well, I have a better code of values now—my intellect is number one, my physical well-being is still of some concern, but of much lesser concern; it's in its proper place. Bodybuilding should be an adjunct to your life, not the reason for it. In fact, if I had to go back and do it over, I would have become a doctor."

Mike was a good friend and, in my humble opinion, one of the brightest minds to have ever entered the world of professional body-building. He had been a pre-med student at the University of Maryland with plans to become a doctor prior to his bodybuilding career catching fire. And because of his studies in organic chemistry, physics, and physiology, he had brought a wealth of science knowledge to bear on his training and nutritional practices. From his vantage point that day he believed not only that he had devoted a disproportionate amount of time to his muscle-building pursuits over the decades, but also that his doing so had caused him to forsake other human pursuits, such as the full cultivation of his intellect and even spiritual cultivation (which he defined as that part of a person which allows him to know himself; i.e., that which he really is).

"Physical training of the type required to win the Olympia demands such physical energy and sustained preoccupation that one is literally forced to shelve one's spiritual and intellectual needs for a long period of time," he said. "I'm not sure it's worth it. When I begin to feel myself losing touch with my center—my spiritual self—I really feel out of sorts and don't enjoy life nearly as much, even though I'm getting in my best physical condition."

"How can you tell when this is occurring?" I asked.

"I can tell when I'm losing this touch with my centering because I just don't enjoy things that I ordinarily enjoy, things which really enrich life for me, like music, reading certain kinds of books. Even emotional relationships become rather tepid at this point, and I've come to discover over the years that the secret in really living a happy life is balance."

Over our coffee that morning we talked about a good many things as was so often the case with Mike. In time the subject returned to exercise, and the general lack of success that many people experience who religiously go to the gym every day. By this point in time Mike had been a personal trainer for two years and through studying his clients' responses to resistance training carefully he had already concluded that most people that he observed training by themselves in the gym were exercising too long and far too frequently. Indeed, he noted that the results of his clients, who trained for short periods of time and far less frequently, were often markedly better. Mike confessed that he had grown frustrated with the ritualistic approach to exercise that most people had embraced, with its tacit implication that if one embraced the "fitness lifestyle" and spent as much time as possible exercising, success would inevitably follow.

"Almost 99.9 percent of all bodybuilders—in fact 99.9 percent of most people—do everything that they do because other people do it," he said. "They do what they do out of convention, imitation, tradition, and outright fear—fear of being 'different.' Rather than risk disapproval or alienation from the group, they completely go along and do what they see others doing—not knowing why it's done, even if it's going to be productive."

After a sip from his coffee Mike elaborated on his point. "I asked a guy in the gym the other day if he knew how to properly use the piece of exercise equipment he was on, thinking I might be able to help him. But the guy waved me off and said, 'I kinda, sorta know how to use it.'"

Mike raised his hands skyward.

"What do you do? This guy and hundreds more like him are going to end up hurting themselves because they don't want to take even one minute to think about an activity that presumably is quite important to them."

He then asked me why, in my opinion, the National Aeronautics Space Administration (NASA) had been so successful over the decades in their quest to send men to the moon and bring them back safely to Earth again. Before I could respond Mike answered his own question.

"NASA has been so spectacularly successful not because they just *kinda, sorta* knew what they were doing, but because they had a firm intellectual grasp of a valid theory of space travel. They had the specific-appropriate knowledge necessary to successfully complete their missions and, as a result, they succeeded."

He paused before continuing.

"The specific-appropriate knowledge necessary for human beings to succeed in anything is available if they just do a little research and think logically about the endeavor they're engaged in. The way most people approach fitness, however, is anything but logical; for the most part they passively accept rituals regarding fitness that have been passed down from generation to generation, or the word of celebrities who know nothing about the requirements of productive exercise. The approach of most people to fitness is tantamount to taking a blind leap into the dark."

I agreed and we further speculated that it didn't have to be that way. Indeed, as Mike saw it, "if NASA can succeed with its space missions—which is an enormously complex goal requiring abstract theoretical knowledge of physics, electronics, astronomy, engineering, and mathematics—you can't tell me we can't succeed with each one of our 'missions to the gym' here on Earth."

He had a point. And yet in looking around our country then and now, it would appear that, unlike NASA and its success in space travel, most people are still failing rather than succeeding in their gym missions within our health and fitness universe. Witness, for example, the number of people who enter the fitness industry each year with fat loss as their primary goal—and yet how few of these people ever achieve it. This is beyond puzzling. We know medically what constitutes fat cells; we further know that if human beings overconsume foodstuffs that any amount taken in beyond what is required to fuel one's vital life processes is converted to fat. And we also know that people with eating disorders who eat very little or those who choose to eat nothing at all end up losing body fat at an alarming rate (as well as their health!). If it were not true that eating less resulted in fat loss then medical conditions such as anorexia nervosa could not exist. But for some reason there exists a majority of people seeking to lose fat who simply fail to connect the dots here and instead are always on the lookout for alternatives to eating less—and one of the more popular alternatives that has been brought forth in this regard is exercise.

The belief is that if one engages in physical activity (i.e., exercise) as often as possible one will lose body fat. And there has been no shortage of people who have employed this alternative method to eating less for several decades now and yet, unless this approach is combined with a reduction in energy consumption (i.e., a food intake that is less than what is required to maintain one's present body weight), little to no difference is ever noted. Could it be that the "exercise it off" approach isn't really as viable an alternative to eating less as we've been led to believe? I would submit that this is, indeed, the case and that the number of people who are now beginning to see through the misty half-truths propagated by the fitness industry is on the rise.

Indeed, as far back as August 2009 *Time* magazine featured a cover story with the provocative headline: "Exercise Won't Make You Thin."[1] To my knowledge, this marked the first official shot over the bow of the fitness industry and revealed some intriguing reasons why many people were beginning to question much of what they thought they knew about exercise and its effects on weight loss, as well as on their health. These reasons have only multiplied in the years since that article was first published. Despite the fact that millions of North Americans in an earnest attempt to lose body fat have been racking up the miles on their treadmills and/or heading out onto the roads for their daily runs, a review of the relevant literature regarding exercise and weight loss reveals that the oft prescribed three-to-five hours per week of moderate to vigorous exercise actually has little or no impact on weight loss.[2]

Even more surprising, researchers from Montreal's McGill University, along with researchers from the University of Toronto, have conducted studies in which they concluded that exercise, per se, could actually be *fattening*![3] In this instance the researchers measured the blood insulin levels of their subjects and noted that insulin levels remained much higher in their obese subjects for well over an hour after they had finished exercising. This caused the researchers to conclude that the bodies of the more obese subjects were able to take glucose out of their bloodstreams and store it as glycogen and, then, when the cells that were emptied of glycogen were replenished, the surplus glycogen was stored as fat.

EXERCISE AND NOTHINGNESS

Quite apart from the news that exercise can have very little effect on fat loss is the fact that exercise may not have *any* effect on certain people at all; that is to say, that a person may not get stronger or improve his or her endurance as a result of engaging in an exercise program.[4] This is an important point to remember, particularly when a celebrity, personal trainer, or magazine article indicates that "you too" can experience the same miraculous transformation that a particular athlete or celebrity is said to have experienced from his or her particular workout program. At best, whatever is being advocated may only work for a small number of people, or even just for the one who happens to be extolling its virtues. At worst, it may not work at all and could actually set you back a step or two.

Once one understands this fact a question automatically arises: if exercise only yields a benefit of somewhere between "0" and "very little" for a certain percentage of the population, then why are so many people willingly devoting hundreds of hours per month to such an enterprise for such a potentially miniscule-to-nonexistent return on their time and energy investment? This question is particularly pertinent given that science has revealed that only a handful of minutes a week of exercise has been shown to stimulate the body to produce whatever benefits exercise can bestow—if the level of muscular work during the exercise session is demanding enough. While we will explore this in greater detail later, one example should suffice.

Researcher Jamie Timmons, a professor of systems biology at Heriot-Watt University in Edinburgh, made headlines throughout the United Kingdom when the result of his eight-year study revealed that a mere three minutes (you read that correctly—three minutes) of muscularly demanding exercise per week was the equivalent of exercise sessions that traditionally had lasted hours. According to an article in the *Daily Mail*:

> So far their tests on hundreds of unfit middle-aged volunteers in Britain and Canada over the past eight years have shown those three minutes of exercise a week deliver the same significant health improvements as can be achieved through hours in the gym or on the running track.[5]

Let that sink in for a moment. And lest the reader think that this is but an isolated example, it should be noted that similar conclusions have also been reached by other researchers in England and Canada,[6] which means that the fact that it's no longer necessary for one to exercise for hours each week is now rather well-settled. Nevertheless, despite such exciting breakthroughs in exercise science, the industry of exercise still remains cluttered with many myths belonging to an older health and fitness paradigm.

Much to my surprise when I embarked on my study of exercise over 20 years ago, almost every conclusion that I had been led to believe about exercise when I began my research would now seem to be if not false, at least faulty. For example, I've learned that partaking in daily physical activity does *not* prevent heart disease nor slow its eventuality. In addition, exercise in itself has virtually no effect on one's longevity. Even more perplexing, it seems that one can be healthy without necessarily being fit and, conversely, one can be tremendously fit and not be very healthy. The reality of the matter is that exercise can *sometimes* be beneficial for *some* people. It is, then, by no means a panacea.

I concede that the above reads as though I'm pouring cold water on the fires of many people's enthusiasm for exercise. However, given how exercise has been so overhyped throughout the years, a dampening of our misplaced enthusiasm might not be such a bad thing. Indeed, I submit that it is only by having a realistic lay of the land up front—that is to say, by first clearly understanding the facts regarding what exercise can and cannot do, before one embarks upon one's exercise journey—that one can know if one's fitness destination is achievable or even if the journey is worth the time investment to embark on at all.

The fact that exercise has limitations isn't discussed much. We certainly don't read articles about "the limitations of exercise" within the pages of the nation's leading fitness magazines, nor is the topic even so much as broached by the various leaders and authorities within the fitness industry itself. Indeed, we're led to believe that the sky is the limit in terms of what one can accomplish in terms of one's health, fitness, and appearance if one puts one's mind to the task and exercises diligently and frequently enough. As proof, we are offered up the incredible physical accomplishments of the world's premiere athletes; the incredible bodies of fitness models, movie, and television celebrities; and the shiny, sinewy physiques displayed on late-night television infomercials. And yet the very fact that these people stand out so much from the norm is the very reason why they were selected to play their particular sports and appear in the product ads in the first place; i.e., they are anomalies in regard to how most people's bodies respond to the stimulus of exercise. Were they not exceptions, then their performance and appearance wouldn't be so striking to us.

ACTIVITY AND HEALTH

So if exercise in and of itself has a transformative effect only on a select few, is devoting so much time to performing a great deal of physical activity at least good for our health? That has certainly been the general belief since 1953, when the English medical journal *Lancet* published a study on British transit workers whose jobs were either sedentary or active.[7] The researchers contrasted both the volume and severity of coronary heart disease that was present among London bus drivers and bus conductors. They noted that the bus drivers, whose jobs only required them to sit and drive their buses, had a much higher incidence of coronary disease than did the bus conductors who routinely had to bound up and down the stairs within double-decker buses to collect fares. The researchers concluded that since the more physically active people in the study had less coronary disease than their less physically active counterparts, they had less coronary disease *because* they *were* more physically active. It would seem a logical conclusion. However, what the study actually revealed was a reversal of cause and effect. The bus drivers who were examined were found to have had a higher risk of heart disease before they began their sedentary jobs and thus selected jobs that required less activity. By contrast, the bus conductors who were examined were at a lower risk for coronary disease before selecting jobs that required more physically demanding work. Being sedentary, then, did not produce heart disease so much as having this condition caused people with this disease not to opt to engage in jobs that required high levels of physical activity. Not surprisingly, this study, the first of its kind, has been considered flawed by critics, but the publication of this technical paper in a scientific journal served to have an impact on medical doctors, who saw its conclusions as a means (higher physical activity) of staving off heart disease and, thus, the recommendation to "be more active" has been with us ever since.

Certainly, physical activity is important, particularly in staving off a loss of muscle and the strength that goes with it. A certain amount of exercise, then, may help to prevent or slow the loss of muscle in our species and, in some instances, even restore what we have lost. This is certainly no small accomplishment, as not only is a weaker body unable to operate at peak efficiency (i.e., optimal functional ability), but the health of that body also suffers, as the metabolic pathways responsible for our health will deteriorate right along with the muscles in which they reside. Indeed, many of the health problems the people experience as they age are tied in with the long-term metabolic problems that attend the loss of muscle. How much muscle does the average person lose as he or she ages? According to some studies, human muscle mass can decrease by nearly 50 percent between the ages of 20 and 90.[8] However, like everything involving our biology, we can only improve our muscular mass and strength up to a genetically mediated limit. Performing more exercise beyond this limit does not appear to drive up higher levels of adaptation.

Additionally, while there most certainly are benefits that can result from having our muscles perform metabolically demanding work, there are also problems that attend doing *any* form of physical activity on a regular basis, and these problems must be weighed in the balance against the alleged health and fitness benefits of the type of activity in which one is engaging so as to determine if the end truly justifies the means. I want to make a distinction here for the sake of clarity; I'm not saying that being completely inactive is desirable or healthy—it's not. But, assuming that one engages in normal day-to-day activities such as walking, climbing stairs, raking leaves, cutting the lawn, shoveling the snow, gardening, etc., your normal activity levels are (for the most part) looked after. However, the type of *supplemental* physical activity (commonly referred to as "exercise") that one chooses to engage in over and above one's normal day-to-day activities is what can prove to be either helpful or harmful in the long-term.

As an interesting side note, many of us are probably more active on a daily basis than we realize. I have a client who is a peak performance coach. He wears a headset while communicating via teleconference with his clients and he is in the habit of pacing while doing so. He recently clipped on a pedometer to determine how much he walked during the multiple phone consultations he performed in a typical day and was surprised to discover that he had walked over three miles—or 21 miles a week—simply by doing his job on a daily basis.

And while the belief that we should be more active is a common one, acting on that belief can bring with it a host of potential problems that might just outweigh any alleged benefits one might be seeking from doing so.

CHAPTER TWO

EXERCISE AND WEAR & TEAR

You've tweaked your elbow playing golf. Another person has a sore back after helping to lift a sofa. A third person is now icing her knee after a short run. And yet another person has a throbbing shoulder after a day at her job as a checkout clerk at a local grocery store. The common denominator in all of the above scenarios is that movement was involved in the occurrence of each injury, and the reason that such movements eventually lead to such injuries is the fact that all physical activity brings wear and tear to your body; if you perform a little bit of physical activity you will suffer a bit of it, and if you perform a lot of it you will suffer a lot of it. Eventually something's got to give and an inflammation or an injury occurs.

Some of this wear and tear is negligible, particularly if we encounter it while we are young, as during the growth cycle that attends adolescence our bodies typically become stronger with each passing year, our cells regenerate regularly and quickly, and minor damage is dealt with quite easily. However, once we have reached a peak in our physical development, which for most of us occurs in and around the age of 25, our bodies begin a slow but discernable process of degradation; i.e., they no longer repair quite so rapidly nor as efficiently as they once did; minor aches and pains now endure for days when in the past they were absent after 24 hours. This is simply a fact of life and there is a reason for it: up until the beginning of the last century the life expectancy for most members of our species was a rather modest 47 years of age.[1] This meant that by age 25 we had typically passed our DNA along via mating and childbirth, and thus the necessity for the original vessel that housed our DNA to continue to output significant amounts of energy in order to rapidly and continuously repair itself was no longer as important (from our DNA's perspective) as it was prior to this genetic handoff having taken place. Consequently, after the age of 25 the repair process slows down considerably.

OUR ARTHRITIC ANCESTORS

Some who advocate for exercising more frequently do so because they have a rather romantic notion that our ancestors were hearty and healthy *because* they were more physically active on a regular basis than we are presently. And while it may be true that our ancestors were more active than we are, this doesn't mean that they experienced superior health—and certainly not a lower mortality rate. Indeed, the paleontological records indicate that a significant number of our ancestors—perhaps *owing* to their higher activity levels—died an early death after first having to endure decades of severe osteoarthritis.[2] According to some records, from the 1500s to around the year 1800, life expectancy throughout Europe fell to somewhere between 30 and 40,[3] and so our ancestors only had to endure their arthritic conditions for perhaps five to 15 years (from age 25 to 40) before death intervened to terminate their lives of chronic pain and compromised mobility. Since the present life expectancy in North America is 80 for men and 84 for women,[4] if we opt to engage in the same volume of activity that led to so much arthritis in our ancestors, we will have to endure this damage and discomfort for more than twice as long as our ancestors ever did, which would reduce the overall quality and enjoyment of our lives considerably.

HINGE JOINTS AND WEAR & TEAR

Every movement we make—from lifting a cup of coffee to going for a walk or a run—can be likened to a rope passing over the edge of a rock in terms of the wear and tear it brings to the joints and connective tissues involved. The elbow and knee joints are classified as "hinge joints" by anatomists and, like the hinges on any door, they will provide the owner with a lifetime of normal use (i.e., a finite number of openings and closings) before they wear out. However, if one adds to this normal rate of wear and tear many more openings and closings as a result of a lot of supplemental physical activity, it doesn't require a postgraduate degree in mathematics to ascertain that those joints are going to wear out that much quicker. For example, going for a modest bicycle ride, a seemingly innocuous activity, requires an average of (give or take) some 10,000 revolutions of the bicycle pedals, representing an additional 10,000 openings and closings of the hinge joints in the knees. Think of how quickly the hinges on your front door would wear out if you routinely opened and closed them 10,000 times (over and above their normal daily use) and did this three, four, or even seven days a week over many months and years. As we've seen, the repair process of the body typically diminishes markedly once we have exited our twenties, with the result that we oldsters enjoy no special immunity from such supplemental wear and tear and, consequently, those who opt to engage in such an activity are putting themselves on a fast track to arthritis and knee replacement surgery.

AEROBICS: DAMAGE VS. BENEFIT

Problems such as the ones indicated above can be exacerbated by activities such as walking, jogging, and cycling, which are typically performed at a lower intensity for longer periods of time, thus resulting in many more thousands of openings and closings of the hinge joints in the knees. For joggers and runners wear and tear is a real concern, but only one of the many problems they face whenever they engage in the performance of their favorite form of exercise. A survey of records of 1,650 amateur runners over a two-year period revealed 19 different injuries to the knee, 22 to the foot, 13 to the lower leg, five to the upper leg, eight to the hip, and four to the lower back, as well as other painful injuries to each area that weren't diagnosed specifically.[5] Decades ago, the cardiologist Henry Solomon wrote a book entitled *The Myth of Exercise*, and within its pages he made some rather (for the time) startling points about the running and jogging craze that was just then starting to mushroom across North America:

> Running injuries are especially common because of the punishing force your body has to take. The impact on each jogging step is two to three times your body weight. On average, your feet will strike the ground 800 to 1,000 times per mile. . . . Exposed to such

stress, it's no wonder that muscular and skeletal injuries happen so often.[6]

Based upon Dr. Solomon's calculations above, a 150-pound runner would accumulate 120 tons of force for every mile he or she runs. However, when Dr. Solomon wrote these words he didn't realize that he was already up against a large industry that would only continue to grow larger with each passing year. At the forefront of the industry was another doctor, Kenneth Cooper, who would become known as the father of the "aerobics" movement (indeed, Cooper was the man who minted the very term). While Solomon focused on cardiology and would go on to serve as the senior medical advisor to the American College of Cardiology, Cooper focused on promoting aerobic exercise and, according to Forbes online magazine, has done rather well with it, becoming the chairman of no fewer than "nine health companies under the Cooper Aerobics umbrella, which includes The Cooper Institute, a nonprofit research education center, [with] 700 employees and revenue totaling $65 million."[7]

Despite having considerable skin in the game, even Cooper would eventually concede that 60 to 70 percent of all runners are hurt badly enough each year that they are required to cut back or stop their running programs completely.[8] Think about that percentage figure—60 to 70 percent—that means that only 30 percent of those who select running as their preferred method of exercise will come out of this activity unscathed after 12 months.

Dr. Solomon further made the point that running was particularly hard on most women, owing to the fact that a woman's center of gravity (where the most force is experienced by the body) is located between her hip bones (a man, by contrast, has his center of gravity located between his waist and chest), which makes women much more susceptible to injuries of the pelvis as a result of running. The naturally wider pelvis of women, which is necessary for childbirth, causes their femurs to descend in an inward angle from the hips, thus placing a disproportionate stress on the inside of their knee joints when running.[9]

The problems associated with endurance activities such as running and cycling don't end with wear and tear and impact trauma. A major health problem where ultra-endurance athletes enjoy no special immunity as a result of their activity is heart disease. According to the online journal *American Medical News*, "Too much endurance running, cycling might weaken the heart."

> While research shows that moderate physical activity improves wellness, studies indicate that too much exercise, particularly extreme endurance events, such as ultra-marathons, can have adverse cardiovascular effects, says a report in the June issue of *Mayo Clinic Proceedings*. . . . The cardiovascular problems that can result from repeated endurance exercise include atrial and ventricular arrhythmias, coronary artery calcification and diastolic dysfunction, the report said.[10]

In checking the June 2012 edition of the *Mayo Clinic Proceedings* we further learn that:

> Over months to years of repetitive injury, this process, in some individuals, may lead to patchy myocardial fibrosis, particularly in the atria, interventricular septum, and right ventricle, creating a substrate for atrial and ventricular arrhythmias. Additionally, long-term excessive sustained exercise may be associated with coronary artery calcification, diastolic dysfunction, and large-artery wall stiffening.[11]

Solomon offered two enlightening definitions on fitness and cardiovascular health that, once understood, go a long way in explaining the confusion that has arisen over these two terms, some even going so far as to consider them synonyms. With regard to fitness, Solomon defined it as "your ability to do physical activity or to perform physical work, a measure of your functioning capacity. It does not reflect the presence or absence of disease and implies nothing about the actual health of your arteries or your heart."[12] Cardiovascular health, on the other hand, refers to "the absence of disease of the heart and blood vessels, not to the ability of an individual to do a certain amount of physical work. Your overall cardiac health is determined by the condition of various heart structures, including the heart muscle, the valves, the special cardiac tissues that carry electrical impulses, and the coronary arteries."[13]

Solomon disagreed that the health of the coronary arteries was the basis for the claims that vigorous exercise was necessary to maintain them, believing that the majority of improvement in one's functional capacity has more to do with its effect on peripheral muscle cells that learn how to extract oxygen more efficiently from the blood, rather than from any improvement in the functioning of the heart. He quoted Dr. George Sheehan (who was a strong advocate for running) as saying:

> You might suspect from the emphasis on cardiopulmonary fitness that the major effect of training is on the heart and lungs. Guess again. Exercise does nothing for the lungs; that has been amply proved. . . . Nor does it especially benefit your heart. Running, no matter what you have been told, primarily trains and conditions the muscles.[14]

And while running may not directly benefit the heart, there is, as we've seen, some strong evidence that it can damage it.

Additionally, though the dangers of low-intensity exercises such as marathon running can be considerable, a need exists nevertheless to preserve our muscular strength and ability in order to function as best as we can as we get older. But what should we do? After all, if we don't do *something* to preserve the strength and functional capacity of our muscles we will become progressively weaker to the point where even the attempt to operate our limbs can become problematic.

To this end a good many of us will try to square this physiological requirement for the preservation of our muscular strength with our psychological desire to socialize. And for this to happen the type of exercise that we choose to perform cannot be too demanding, or else it would negatively impact our capacity to socialize (after all, the intense lactic acid burn and labored breathing that often attends demanding muscular work really doesn't present an ideal environment in which to conduct discourse). As a result, most people will simply opt to partake in exercise programs that are comprised of low-intensity physical activity that then must be carried on for longer periods (for upwards of an hour in most instances) in order to fatigue their muscles to any meaningful degree. As a consequence, such people rack up huge amounts of wear and tear in the process of trying to synchronize their exercise sessions with their desire to be social.

A preference for low-energy output activity has been prevalent almost since the fitness industry's inception. Runners are quite often seen running in pairs or groups, talking to each other as they attempt to increase their distances, and mistakenly believing that they are increasing their health as they do so. I've known many runners who have come to my training facility over the years and when I try to save their joints by pointing out that they don't need to be incurring such wear and tear in order to be healthy or fit, I am invariably told that they are addicts of the "runner's high," a not-always-occurring but legendary feeling of euphoria that attends the activity of running. However, one can rationalize almost any activity (no matter how damaging it is to the body) by saying it makes one feel good. It is the standard response offered by most addicts to justify their unhealthy addictions.

CHAPTER THREE

STRESS, INSULIN, AND THE NON-RESPONDER

Two of your friends are stressed out. One of them seeks to alleviate her stress by consuming what has popularly been called "comfort foods"—items such as cookies, ice cream, potato chips—that are quickly broken down and converted to glucose by the body. The rising levels of glucose make her feel less irritable, less edgy, and more relaxed. Your other friend seeks to relieve his stress by going to the gym. He makes a point of working out every day for at least an hour. Such physical activity temporarily takes his mind off of his problems, burns through the glucose stores in his muscles, and releases certain hormones that make him feel better. These scenarios reveal one problem (stress) with two common approaches to dealing with it (eating and exercise). However, it could be that both of these approaches are doing more harm than good.

Let us consider the case of your first friend: her consumption of foodstuffs that are easily and rapidly converted into glucose can be disastrous as it creates a situation whereby insulin has to be secreted in greater quantities in order to deal with the increasing levels of sugar in her bloodstream. Excess glucose invariably gets converted to bodyfat, and her chronically high insulin levels can often leave the lining of many of the cells within her body inflamed. This cellular inflammation can grow and spread throughout her body, until it becomes systemic. And here is where real health problems can begin, as inflammation on the surface of cells will be mortared by cholesterol (which is all that cholesterol is—mortar to patch inflamed areas on cells). When cholesterol levels become high, physicians will often prescribe a class of drugs known as statins to lower their patients' high cholesterol levels. However, this only treats the *symptom* (the higher cholesterol levels) but leaves the *source* of the rising cholesterol levels (the cellular inflammation) untouched. As a result, many of us continue to live—with or without statins—with chronically inflamed cells. For such people, engaging in exercise of any stripe is definitely *not* a healthy thing to do, as exercise can also produce an inflammatory effect in various cells within the body, which will only compound the problem. For these people it is better not to exercise at all until they have corrected the lifestyle issues that have produced their chronically inflamed states. To throw exercise into the mix at this point would be the equivalent of throwing gasoline on a fire in the hope of extinguishing it.

The same would apply to the second friend in the above scenario; even if his genetics were such that he responded favorably to the stimulus of exercise, if he were truly under stress and seeking to relieve his stress through exercise, any results he might have stimulated would be prevented from being produced as a result of an overabundance of stress hormones such as cortisol that his system would already be awash with. If by chance either of the two people in our above example liked to drink and smoke, then both of them would have not only chronically inflamed systems, but systems that are working overtime trying to put out the numerous internal fires that their poor lifestyle choices keep setting on a daily basis. In this context, adding the stress of exercise to an already stressed-to-capacity physiology could be the proverbial straw that breaks the camel's back.

Knowing this, the popular conception of exercise being a "stress reliever" is revealed to be without physiologic foundation. According to the late medical doctor and stress research pioneer Hans Selye, stress is *everything* in your life and only death can liberate you from its influence. Consequently, you can't relieve stress simply by changing its form. If you want to diminish the amount of cellular stress that your body is under, then back away from the potato chips, the refined sugars, the flour, the excessive intake of grains and cereals, the soft drinks, the alcohol, the tobacco, and all of the other agents that are causing your physiology to work overtime in order to tamp out the cellular (and systemic) inflammation. Doing so will do infinitely more to reduce your stress levels in a very literal sense than knocking off 45 minutes on a treadmill, taking an aerobics class, punching a heavy bag, or lifting weights. How such activities have acquired a reputation as being stress relievers is that engaging in them causes one to focus on these activities—rather than whatever personal issues had been consuming their psyches. Worry can be defined as mental stress, so any distraction serves the purpose of temporarily getting your mind off of the subject or event that is consuming or otherwise bothering you. But mental angst is not the same as metabolic stress, which is a physiologic cause and effect scenario. In some instances, mental angst can result in psychosomatic disorders if the problem that is vexing you is not faced, dealt with, and resolved. Indeed, mental worries can in some cases lead to ulcers, which is a physiological event. But if we are talking about a stressed physiology, doing things that will only exacerbate such a condition, such as overeating or overexercising, is a step in the wrong direction. Don't misunderstand me—exercise can help to reduce cellular inflammation, but only to a degree that can easily be overwhelmed by one's continuing to consume foodstuffs and ingest agents that keep one's system in a perpetually inflamed (stressed) state.

DUMPING GLYCOGEN

In the quest to reduce metabolic stress, not all exercises are created equal. A certain type of exercise can actually serve in some capacity to reduce cellular inflammation somewhat, but only if it is performed in a manner that taps the muscle fibers that store the most glycogen (polymers of glucose or blood sugar). These fibers, known as Fast-Twitch fibers, are typically the fibers of last resort for your body to employ during a given exercise. If the load placed on working muscles is great enough, your body will cycle through all (or most) of its three classes of muscle fibers (Slow-Twitch, Intermediate-Twitch, and Fast-Twitch) to keep your muscles working at such a high level of effort. If the energy level your muscles are outputting is high enough, your body will recruit most of these fibers instantaneously; if the energy level you are outputting is low, then your body will eventually recruit them over a longer period of time. Either method will take you to this destination; the latter simply takes longer to get there and runs up a greater amount of wear and tear (and hence metabolic inflammation) in the process. But it is important to know that once you tap these glycolytic fibers you are causing them to dump a huge amount of sugar (glycogen) from your muscles, thereby creating empty reservoirs for your circulating blood sugar to refill. Without this glucose evacuation, when you consume foodstuffs that are converted to glucose quickly, insulin must be brought in immediately to help process the rising level of sugar in the bloodstream, but since the muscles (which, along with the liver, store most of the glycogen in the body) are still filled with untapped glycogen, insulin will have no option but to transform the new glucose into additional fat cells, thus making you fatter. Prior to this, however, insulin will first attempt to enter your muscle cells with these glucose molecules but will be denied entry. However, the insulin will keep "scratching at the door" of the muscle cell and this "scratching" is what causes the inflammation on the lining of the cell/s.

This is why popular lower-intensity endurance (or "cardio") exercise can actually be a step in the wrong direction if one is seeking to reduce one's cholesterol levels in any meaningful way. An endurance activity requires an endurance fiber, which happens to be a Slow-Twitch fiber, and Slow-Twitch fibers just happen to store the *least* amount of glycogen of the three classes of muscle fiber, meaning that it takes almost no time for the miniscule amount of glycogen they possess to be emptied and replaced, which leaves one suffering from high cholesterol levels right back where he or she started from prior to performing his or her cardio workout.

And, if a person continues to perform his cardio (i.e., low-energy output, longer duration) exercises frequently enough his body will eventually get the message that the other two fiber types are not required and will send a signal to downsize the unused Intermediate and Fast-Twitch muscle fibers, which are the human body's biggest reservoirs for glucose storage. If this person continues to perform his endurance exercise, these large glucose-storing fibers will continue to diminish in size over time through lack of use, thus giving his person's body no exit from the systemic inflammation, save severe dietary restriction. This is why walking as an exercise really does little to nothing from a health standpoint once one initially adapts to it. While it's true that to a couch potato walking may be a demanding activity at first, his body will adapt quite quickly to this activity (for reasons I'll get to shortly) and, over time, will require less of his higher-order fibers to participate in the activity, landing the walking advocate in the position indicated above.

Again, the single best cure for systemic inflammation and the higher cholesterol levels that attend it is to stop inputting into one's system the materials that are causing the inflammation in the first place. The reduction or elimination of the foodstuffs and exogenous agents that are causing one's system to become inflamed will do more for one's health than any exercise program. Exercise is fine—after you've tended to the lifestyle issues.

EXERCISE & THE NON-RESPONDER

In returning to a point made earlier, it must be remembered that apart from the problems indicated above with regard to exercise and stress, there is also the fact that there exists a percentage of people who, despite their diligence in investing hours, weeks, months, and years in the venture of exercise, will never experience any of the benefits that exercise has the potential to bestow. A study out of Finland revealed that there exists a portion of people who simply *do not respond* to strength training and some people who simply *do not respond* to endurance (aerobic) exercise. There are even those who simply *do not respond* to either. The researchers took 175 sedentary adults and put them on a 21-week exercise program. The subjects were divided into groups that jogged, walked, lifted weights, or combined the three activities. The fitness and muscular strength of the subjects were measured prior to and at the conclusion of the study and, to the surprise of the researchers, the data was all over the board, running from a -8 percent (meaning that some became 8 percent less fit than they were prior to starting the exercise program) to a +42 percent.[1] Some of those who lifted weights became stronger, but some didn't. Some of those who jogged and walked developed more aerobic endurance, but some didn't. In other words, it was revealed that some people respond very well to the stimulus of exercise, but (and this is a big "but") some *do not respond at all* or actually lose ground in terms of their fitness and health.

Jamie Timmons, a professor of systems biology at the Royal Veterinary College in London, in her review of the foregoing study indicated in the

Journal of Applied Physiology that, "there will be millions of humans that cannot improve their aerobic capacity or their insulin sensitivity, nor reduce their blood pressure through exercise."[2] Now if ever there was an "ah-ha!" moment with regard to the fitness industry, surely this was it. Think about the implications of this study for a moment; if you engage in an exercise program—irrespective of whether it is aerobics-based or strength-based, there exists the possibility that the activity you are engaging in will make you less aerobically fit, weaker, or, at best, do nothing for you at all. Now ask yourself why such a landmark study never made it onto the front covers of the nation's fitness magazines. Not one of them carried it. The reason is self-evident: it would have been bad for business.

The results of this study were/are so remarkable that it left many people looking for reasons as to why the conclusion came out the way that it did. In an attempt to look into the matter more thoroughly, *New York Times* writer Gretchen Reynolds contacted Dr. Timmons, a researcher who has studied the role of genetics in exercise response. Reynolds reported the following about her conversation with the good doctor, citing a study conducted by Dr. Timmons to determine who would respond most favorably to endurance exercise. Timmons's study revealed that:

> Researchers accurately predicted who would respond most to endurance exercise training based on the expression levels of 29 different genes in their muscles before the start of the training. Those 29 genes are not necessarily directly associated with exercise response. They seem to have more to do with the development of new blood vessels in muscles; they may or may not have initiated the response to exercise. Scientists just don't know yet.
>
> In other words, this issue is as intricate as the body itself. There is a collection of compelling data that indicate that about half of our aerobic capacity "is genetic," Dr. Timmons wrote in an e-mail. "The rest may be diet," or it could be a result of epigenetics, a complicated process in which the environment (including where you live and what you eat) affects how and when genes are activated. "Or it could be other factors," he said.

Although fewer studies have examined why people respond so variously to strength training, "we have no reason to doubt," he said, "that genetics play a similar role."[3]

It has come more clearly into focus over the years that an individual's physical characteristics are determined more by his or her genetics and lifestyle choices than it is the particular exercise program he or she happens to embrace. Unfortunately, many of the dietary and lifestyle choices that most people make put them on a road to ill health from which no trainer or exercise program can extricate them.

CHAPTER FOUR

EXERCISE—THE NOT-SO-HEALTHY ADDICTION

People who feel the need to exercise frequently will often refer to their exercise sessions as a "healthy addiction." But is it? While the "addiction" component may be accurate, whether such activity is healthy is open to considerable debate.

Katherine Schreiber was a young lady who was addicted to exercise and whose story was told within the pages of the *British Medical Journal*:

> By the time KS entered college, her world revolved around the gym. No sooner would she finish a lecture than she would dash to the campus fitness center. She would feel anxious if she missed a workout and would go no matter how tired or busy she was. . . . She lost many friendships and career opportunities because she was barely available outside her exercise schedule. By the time she was 26 years old, KS had weathered two herniated discs and a stress fracture and had persistent exhaustion.[1]

The paper went on to state that, "Although exercise addiction is not officially classified as a mental health disorder, it is characterized by similar negative effects on emotional and social health as other addictions."[2] This is a phenomenon that the author of this book experienced himself during his first four years of working out. Certain family gatherings were given a miss because I *had to* work out—which at that time I was doing seven days a week. Looking back on that part of my life I can only shake my head in bewilderment and be grateful that I was somehow able to pull myself out of that psychological tailspin. But for many people who are stuck in the middle of that vortex, escape not only seems impossible, but also something that they are overtly hostile to the very suggestion of. Escape? From something that's good for you? Who would opt for that? But what if, as in the example of Katherine Schreiber above, such frequent exercise is not so good for you?

Exercise, it might be said, has two sides, with one half of it yielding the potential to do good and the other half yielding the potential to do harm. The good, obviously, lies in the potential for exercise to stimulate your body to become stronger, and to preserve muscle fibers that might otherwise be left to decondition and atrophy.

Indeed, exercise can give our bodies a strong impetus to retain (or, in the case of sarcopenia, reclaim) muscle fibers and the multiple metabolic pathways contained within them, which will serve to preserve (and often enhance) one's functional ability. In addition, we've seen that the type of exercise that accomplishes this (high-energy output exercise) also produces the event of emptying the glycogen stores within our muscle fibers, which can stave off potentially health-threatening conditions such as type II diabetes, high blood pressure, arterial plaque, and heart disease.

However, the potential for exercise to do harm also exists, and that potential lies in the fact that most approaches to exercise (particularly ones that also seek to tap Fast-Twitch muscle fibers) can subject our muscles, joints, and connective tissues to a fair degree of trauma. To be clear, not all exercise approaches are equal in either their good and bad qualities. Some (such as resistance training), can deliver a large portion of the good, with only a little bit of the bad component; other approaches (such as running, leaving aside the fact that it only recruits and stimulates the muscles of the lower extremities) can likewise deliver a large amount of the good, but it's packaged with a large amount of the bad as well. The millions of steps taken over a career of running or jogging, the hundreds of thousands of rotations of limbs during swimming, and a similar number of opening and closing of knee joints during cycling can all add up to trouble over time.

And while this should almost be self-evident, many trainees seem to believe that since they have yet to experience any such negative effects from their exercise sessions that they won't experience any such effects in the future. This is a pitfall that is unfortunately all too common among athletes and their coaches, as athletes are often told that they can't be active enough; that their competitors may be doing more than they are; and that if they wish to excel in their chosen sport, then they will need to equal (or better yet, exceed) what their fellow competitors are doing.

SKILL TRAINING VS. CONDITIONING TRAINING

The problem with the belief that since no injuries have been experienced yet that this will remain so into the future is that such a "so far, so good" approach only takes into consideration the negative effects that show up immediately during a practice or a game, which typically involves younger athletes whose systems are more prone to rapid recovery and whose injuries mend quickly as part and parcel of the growth cycle that all young people enjoy. It does not take into account the consequences that can come home to roost further down the road when these same athletes become older and their self-repair systems less efficient. I should sidetrack here to mention that exercise—that is, physical activity that is purposefully engaged in to alter some aspect of one's physiology for the better (such as improving one's strength, muscular endurance, or health)—is not the same as physical activity that is performed simply to perfect a skill set that is required for a particular sport. The latter falls under the category of motor learning or neural-muscular phenomenon and requires little energy but a high volume of repetition in order to properly lay down the neuromuscular pathways that will allow one to achieve the necessary dexterity one requires for a particular skill (from dribbling a basketball and hitting a golf ball to stickhandling a puck and throwing a football). Exercise performed to induce biological change, by contrast, requires that the trainee attempt to tap as many of his or her muscle fibers as possible, which results in an outputting of a large amount of energy. In other words, exercise that is performed for the purpose of increasing one's strength and metabolic health has to be demanding if it is to warrant the body producing a change that in itself requires a considerable energy investment, such as the creation of more muscle tissue that it must then innervate and supply with energy on an ongoing basis. Skill training, by contrast, requires practice—and lots of it—in order for an athlete to achieve some degree of mastery. Skill training almost can't be overdone for the reason that it's not particularly demanding (which is why it can be performed for so long and so frequently), along with the fact that one simply can't achieve mastery of a skill without practice. However, the more demanding the training, the greater the need for the body to rest, recover, and repair itself. And the recovery and repair processes are two distinct and separate processes that aren't completed immediately after a workout, game, or practice. It can (as we shall see in later chapters) take upwards of several days or more.

A HOCKEY STORY

To better illustrate this, I should mention that I have supervised several studies on the issue of recovery from exercise involving hockey players, and each of these has made it crystal clear that once the hockey season begins, any demanding form of exercise (such as resistance training) added into a player's schedule is a step in the wrong direction—and this is true even for players in their teenage years. I mention this because it is currently in fashion for coaches to have their players engage in what they term "off ice training," wherein the players, in addition to their games and practices, are encouraged (or often expected) to participate in vigorous exercise during the days that they are away from the rink. This is done blindly, however, without the coaches even being aware of what effect the games and practices have on their players' physiologies.

What first drew my attention to this matter was when one of my trainers, Blair Wilson, signed with a junior "A" hockey club in our area. He was an excellent hockey player who was in top condition as a result of a schedule of resistance training that he had engaged in during the off-season. However, as the hockey season was now rapidly approaching, Blair became curious as to how often he could engage in his strength training workouts once the season started, or what effect the added activity of practices and games would have on his existing levels of strength and muscle mass. His chief concern was that he didn't want to lose the muscle mass and strength that he had built up, as it was his wish to remain as strong as possible for each and every game. At the time neither of us had any idea what effects his twice-weekly hockey practices (and two games a week) would have on his body composition. Then there was the matter of what activities the coaches would have his team doing within the practices themselves; i.e., would they be doing "suicides" (that is, having the players skate in sprint-like fashion up and down the rink repeatedly—a very demanding form of exercise), or would they be focusing instead on skill training drills such as passing, shooting, and puck handling? Then there were the games themselves, with every player expected to play each and every shift "all out." Consequently, a game or practice would certainly be the equal of a very demanding exercise session, and all of these factors in and of themselves would place an incredible demand upon a player's recovery ability.

At that time my training facility had a very sophisticated body composition-testing machine called a BodPod (the Mayo Clinic presently has one in each of its three facilities) that we used for monitoring compositional changes in our clients' muscle mass and body fat levels. Blair and I decided that we should check his body composition prior to his very first practice at the start of the season and then check it every day throughout the season. That way we could see if he was gaining or losing muscle mass as the season progressed. I knew from previously testing subjects who performed demanding workouts that the immediate post-workout effect on body composition was a drop in lean mass, as energy had left the muscle and often there was minor damage that had occurred. After several days of rest, however, it was consistently noted that the diminished lean mass would begin to track back up until it reached the level it had been prior to the exercise session and then, after a few more days of rest and recovery, it would typically exceed that previous level. Tracking Blair's body composition on a daily basis allowed us a means to discern when his body had recovered sufficiently so that we could add his strength training workouts into the mix and allow him to either continue to build his strength or (at the very least) maintain his strength and muscle mass as the season progressed.

Blair agreed to keep a journal so that we would know what he did in practice and then, as a result of our daily compositional testing, we could learn what effect these activities had on his body. What we found out almost immediately from the daily testing of his body composition was that Blair couldn't engage in supplemental training at all. From September (when the season started) until mid December he lost over six pounds of muscle tissue. The reason being that his coaches had him performing two practices a week, which were then increased to three, and then he had to play one or two games every weekend. This was the equivalent of performing several "all-out" workouts a week—for four months straight! So even the idea of a maintenance workout would have simply represented a "piling on" in terms of additional energy output and damage to his muscles and would have caused him to lose even more muscle. This was important to note, as a reduction in muscle mass means a reduction in muscle power, strength, and the ability of an athlete's body to resist injury. But quite apart from the damage that occurs to muscles during a workout is the fact that an athlete's muscles are weaker after a workout. Consequently, if a muscle that is operating at 100 percent peak efficiency will tear when subjected to 100 pounds of force, that means that an athlete is safe in encountering up to 99 pounds of force. But if that muscle becomes smaller and weaker as a result of a workout, then that number could drop down to 60—and the athlete's chance of injury would increase by 33.3 percent. In other words, the athlete who engages in supplemental training during his competitive season could well be setting himself up for an injury that would not have occurred if he did not engage in the supplemental training.

As the season progressed, Blair began to run composition testing on other teammates and noted the exact same phenomenon occurring. Once we understood the full effect that practices and games had on an athlete's body (i.e., a weakening effect), it only stood to reason that no coach should want to weaken his players prior to sending them out onto the ice to compete, but rather he should want to do everything in his power to send out players who were fully recovered and at their strongest. Given the depleting effect that practices and games have on a player's physiology, what became evident is that the hockey players need more recovery time in between practices and games—not more exercise.

I grant that this information flies directly in the face of most coaching practices. For example, if a hockey team appears lethargic and slow in the third period of a game, the coaches' typical solution is to work their players very hard in the very next practice. If the team plays poorly, the coaches usually don't consider that the players might not have recovered from the previous game that they played, or their last practice, and so they prescribe a physically demanding activity, such as "suicides," that just simply augers a deeper hole into the players' energy reserves. Eventually, if they're lucky, the players will get sick or incur a minor injury—as a sickness or a minor injury then brings much needed rest into the players' schedule. If they're unlucky, the player will suffer a career-ending injury, an injury that was preventable if proper attention had been paid to the magnitude of the toll that hard high-energy output practices and games take on a player's physiology. If such high-energy output practices are going to continue—and presumably they will because you won't change coaching beliefs overnight, particularly when a very lucrative "off ice conditioning" business has insinuated itself into the very ethos of the sport (I know of one hockey school that charges players $10,000 a week for instruction and another $3,000 a week for food!)—then it may be incumbent upon the athlete to do his best to try and build up as much of a muscular cushion as he can during the off-season, because he's simply going to lose a good part of it once the season starts.

The minor leagues of most sports take their direction from the professional teams, not realizing that most professional sports teams enjoy a success and profile that are far more a result of the genetic composition of their players than the supplemental training approach in which the players often engage. Quite clearly whenever there is money to be made competition becomes thick, with trainers looking for any angle that will get them more clients. Since most athletic trainers are not necessarily great athletes themselves, they can't really offer much to the athlete in terms of improving their skill set for a given sport and, without that angle, they are left with physical conditioning (exercise) as their ticket to bigger paydays. But since every other strength and conditioning coach has the exact same card to play, the aspiring trainer of a professional sports team either has to know the person personally who does the hiring, or he has to offer something that will set his program apart from those of his competitors. And this is why you will see some strength and conditioning coaches having their athletes run with small parachutes strapped to their backs, hitting tires with sledgehammers, climbing ropes, flipping monster truck tires (tires again), and a host of other variations on the resistance training theme (after all, their muscles are contracting against resistance in each instance, or contracting their muscles against drag in the case of the parachute, which is another way of applying resistance to working muscles). Since every trainer is competing with other trainers for a job, if one is lucky enough to get hired as the official strength and conditioning coach of a professional sports team, then his approach is given instant cache, as it is then viewed as the approach that sports teams (or at least a sports team) want and are willing to pay money to trainers to implement for them. Thereafter, the strength and conditioning coach is virtually guaranteed even more clients in the form of aspiring young players (and their parents, who typically foot the bill for their services) who seek similar success. Whether the strength and conditioning coach's methods are the best (or even safe) is seldom looked into very critically. This was particularly evident when three Oregon football players were hospitalized after "enduring a series of grueling strength and conditioning workouts," according to a report out of Oregon.[3] This resulted in the team's strength coach being suspended and the story being picked up nationally.

I recall once being approached by a man who wanted me to train his son who had both the talent and good fortune to be drafted into the Ontario Hockey League (OHL). The OHL is the penultimate rung on the hockey ladder, the last step before a player enters the National Hockey League (NHL). It is absolutely crucial at this stage of a young hockey player's journey that he arrives at his OHL training camp at his absolute physical peak. Not only is an athlete who is in peak strength able to do everything at full power for longer periods of time, but also his chances of getting injured are greatly reduced. I provided the father of this young man with some reading material consisting of independently conducted studies that revealed the dangers of overtraining young athletes, in addition to explaining to him the difference between skill training and conditioning training. I then told him to go home with his son and read the materials and, if after reading the materials, it made sense to the father that his son should train only as often as was required (rather than as often as possible), and devote the remainder of his time to the perfecting of his hockey skills, then I would agree to train him.

Early the next day I received a call from the father indicating that "it all makes perfect sense" and that he wanted to have his son start training with me at my facility right away. Over the course of the first several workouts the young athlete was making excellent progress, but then, for some reason, his progress began to slow down and then it ceased altogether. I asked the young man if he was doing anything else that might be interfering with his recovery from his workouts at my facility. He informed me that after the first several weeks of his training—in which his strength was increasing each week—his father told him that he didn't think he was "doing enough" at the gym (the workouts I had him performing were shorter in duration than those advocated by the strength and conditioning coaches of several OHL teams). As a result, right after his son's training session with me, the father would then drive the young man to another personal trainer in town where he would then be trained all over again for one to two more hours. But apparently even this wasn't enough (after all, other athletes who might be in competition with his son for a spot on the team might be doing more still), and so he added into the mix sending his son to a "hockey conditioning specialist" who, at great expense, had the young man skate very hard up and down the length of the ice with a parachute strapped to his back—and also had the boy running several miles a day. I'm sorry to report that the young man went on to have a very mediocre training camp, saw little ice time on the OHL team that drafted him, and never made it to the NHL. A tragic example of the fear of not doing enough sabotaging a player's shot at making the big time.

This attitude of "if a little is good, then more must be better," is not just wrong, it's dangerous. Unfortunately, it is also a very pervasive attitude within our culture. It's not unusual to read about someone taking four times the recommended dose of an over-the-counter medication under the mistaken belief that it will cure one's headache symptoms four times quicker. Unfortunately, it has no heightened beneficial effect in this regard—but taking more than the recommended dose may just burn a hole in one's stomach lining. Similarly, taking in too much sunlight doesn't accelerate the tanning process, but it will result in burning and blisters. And, in a similar vein, too much exercise doesn't make you a stronger athlete, it weakens you—and it doesn't make you healthier. Beyond a certain threshold, doing more exercise simply weakens your immune system and protracts the time it takes for you to recover and grow stronger from your exercise sessions. In my supervising all of the workouts that I have over the years (and to date I've supervised in excess of 70,000 of them) I've never seen an instance where doing more than is required resulted in anything except reduced progress.

PART TWO

EXERCISE—THE OLD PARADIGM

CHAPTER FIVE

RUNNING FOR HEALTH AND FAT LOSS

When most people think of exercise, they picture someone running. So pervasive is this activity that according to the magazine *Running Room* there are 37 million runners in North America.[1] Some run short distances, some run long distances, and others believe that nothing satisfies their quest for exercise quite like a marathon. Running is not only incredibly popular, but it has also been hailed by some over the years as "the king of exercises" and our species' "natural" form of exercise. However, running—even for short distances—can have more than its fair share of problems. In fact, the scientific literature is strongly suggestive that the more time spent in this activity (whether in terms of the amount of minutes devoted to it per session or the number of times one engages in it per week), the greater the health risks you may well encounter. This is particularly true for those who take part in ultra-endurance events such as marathon running. The ultra-endurance athletes have been shown to be much more likely than their less active counterparts to develop a host of serious health ailments, including:

1. Cardiovascular disease[2]
2. Atrial fibrillation[3]
3. Cancer[4]
4. Liver and gallbladder disorders[5]
5. Muscle damage[6]
6. Kidney dysfunction (renal abnormalities)[7]
7. Acute microthrombosis in the vascular system[8]
8. Brain damage[9]
9. Spinal degeneration[10]

The ultra-endurance athletes are also at risk for certain types of germ cell cancers.[11] One study found that those who participated in college athletics for at least five hours a week were 1.66 times more likely to develop prostate cancer than were those who participated less than five hours a week,[12] while another study found that those college athletes who had attained one or more letters in varsity sports had increased mortality from prostate cancer relative to those who had not.[13] And if that isn't enough to give pause to those who are considering upping their weekly quotient of cardio exercise, there is further evidence that exercise that lasts more than several hours and is performed for multiple days in a row can lead to blood poisoning. Researcher Dr. Ricardo Costa from Monash University in Australia conducted a study involving people who participated in extreme endurance events such as 24-hour marathons and concluded that:

> Nearly all of the participants in our study had blood markers identical to patients admitted to hospital with sepsis.[14]

Some might be tempted to conclude that if ultra-endurance exercise yields the potential to be that dangerous, perhaps it would be safer to simply run for shorter distances, such as a 10-kilometer race. Over the years I've lost count of the number of people who have informed me that their goal is to run a 10K. Many believe that running such a race is a good thing to do for their cardiovascular health, while others see it as a marker of sorts to indicate that they've achieved a desired level of endurance fitness. Certainly running a 10K requires a level of endurance fitness, but it does not necessarily require a healthy cardiovascular system, as people have been known to drop dead from heart attacks while running a 10K, indicating that some form of cardiovascular disease was thriving despite all of the preparatory aerobic exercise these people were engaged in.[15]

It must be noted that there is nothing about exercise, per se, that will bestow upon its practitioner a longer life. As psychiatrist Carl Jung pointed out, "Life itself is a disease with a very poor prognosis; it lingers on for years and invariably ends with death." And while life cannot be prolonged by exercise, it can nevertheless be shortened by its absence, which will set into motion a series of events whereby one becomes less mobile and less capable of efficiently processing the energy that is being input into one's system.

And in the event a person chooses to take action to remain as fit and healthy as long as possible, there is one thing he or she should know about fitness and improving one's health, and that is that there exist *limits* to the ultimate levels of development for both fitness and health that simply cannot be transcended. Once one has reached this genetic ceiling, doing more and more of a certain activity will not drive up higher and higher levels of adaptation. This is an important point to keep in mind, particularly if you are one of those people who believes that you have to do more of whatever exercise you happen to be performing in order to make continual progress.

Once people make their peace with the fact that the majority of human beings don't require an ever-increasing amount of physical activity in order to achieve whatever results exercise can bestow, the first objection that comes to the mind of some is, "What about my cardio? Don't I require a more frequent type of training just to keep my cardiovascular system healthy?" As a matter of fact, you don't. As it turns out, you can get the same benefits (in terms of cardiovascular health) from running fast and hard for five to 10 minutes that you can from running more than three hours.[16] It is now well settled that short bursts of high-energy muscular work can provide the same benefits as long, more endurance-oriented exercise.[17] Indeed, in 2012 a study was conducted that compared a group of runners who performed traditional, longer duration runs with a group of runners who did interval training and revealed that both groups achieved virtually the same results in terms of the impact on body composition, resting heart rate, aerobic power, and oxygen uptake.[18] However, there was one difference between the two groups—the interval trainers demonstrated a better peak oxygen uptake (one of the more important indices of endurance) than the runners who ran for hours and hours each week.

For those who believe they have to do a high volume of exercise in order to be fit and healthy, it should be pointed out that performing longer bouts of endurance ("cardio") exercise can actually be bad for you, and has actually been shown to reduce your body's natural ability to fend off upper respiratory infections such as colds and flu, whereas working out with high-energy output effort (which results in a much shorter workout) will actually improve your immune function. This not only reduces the chances of your getting sick but also reduces the severity of any illness that you might develop.[19]

The old paradigm that separated muscular work from cardiovascular work was predicated on the errant belief that muscle tissue was somehow divorced from the heart and blood vessels. It's not. In fact, what most people refer to as "cardio" pertains to the aerobic subsection of human metabolism. And the aerobic subsection resides in the mitochondria, which are located within each of our cells. By far the most mitochondria are located in muscle cells owing to the fact that muscle cells require a lot of energy to function and the mitochondria contain (or at least can produce) a lot of energy onsite for working muscles to use.

MITOCHONDRIA & MUSCLE

There are more mitochondria in our muscles than there are in our bones or skin. When your muscles perform work, the demand for fuel (nutrients delivered through circulating blood) increases to help keep the muscular activity going. The more demanding the muscular work, the more fuel is required, and this requires the aerobic machinery within the cells to be fully engaged. It therefore stands to reason that your heart and blood vessels aren't disengaged when your muscles are working hard and outputting great amounts of energy. In fact, they are involved to a greater degree the more demanding the muscular work is that you are performing. If you are engaged in an activity that isn't very demanding, the need for energy in the form of adenosine triphosphate (ATP) is minimal, and so the krebs cycle that operates within the mitochondria doesn't have to cycle very quickly. However, if you are performing an activity that is very demanding, the need for energy is increased dramatically and the krebs cycle turns very quickly in order to create more ATP.

PERPETUAL AEROBICS

According to the Mayo Clinic, the average resting heart rate for adults is 60 to 100 beats per minute,[20] which means that the human heart contracts somewhere between 86,400 and 144,000 times a day. This is a considerable amount of contractions—the equivalent of the amount of contractions your quadriceps muscle would make if you ran between three and four marathons a day. Now, if you were performing between 86,400 and 144,000 biceps curls a day, do you really think your biceps muscle would require *more* exercise than this on a weekly basis in order to be healthy? Quite the contrary, you would probably think that this was more than enough. Not so, apparently, with many cardio advocates, who strive to add more beats per minute to their cardiac muscle's already considerable workload several days a week. It's clear from the above data that even when you are sleeping you are in fact engaged in "cardio" as your aerobic system is still engaged; i.e., your heart is beating, oxygenated blood is being circulated, and waste products are being removed from active cells. And it follows from this that your aerobic machinery only cranks up from this baseline whenever you perform activities that are more demanding than sleeping. Anything you do involving more demanding muscular activity requires a more rapid transport of oxygenated blood and an increase in the rate of normal systole and diastole. Walking requires more of the aerobic machinery to be engaged than does standing; jogging requires more than walking; running requires more than jogging, and sprinting requires more than running. And so it follows that if you truly wish to maximally engage your cardiovascular system you must perform maximally demanding muscular work.

High-energy output activity amps cardiovascular activity within the body far more effectively than does low-energy output muscular work that is merely carried on for longer periods of time and this is the primary reason that I have no conventional "cardio" machines in my facility. My clients get all the cardio they need from working their muscles in a high-energy output fashion with proper resistance training. Resistance training, performed the way I advocate, requires that a lot of aerobic work take place in order to process the waste products that accrue from hardworking muscles. One of these waste products is lactic acid, which is then converted to the enzyme pyruvate and shuttled into the mitochondria where it is processed aerobically at a very high rate. So your "cardio" is well looked after with a high energy-output resistance training workout. In looking to the animal kingdom, we note an optimized cardiovascular system is essential to every animal species' survival, but there is not one animal species outside of ourselves that you will ever see jog or perform special "cardio" exercises.

McMaster University in Hamilton, Ontario, Canada, has been one of the leading institutions of research in this field and several studies that have been conducted by their physiology department over the years have conclusively established that while low-intensity, less demanding muscular work performed for 90 minutes three times a week will stimulate an improvement in one's aerobic capacity, the same degree of improvement can also be stimulated with four to five 30-second intervals (a total of 2 to 2.5 minutes of muscular work) performed "all out."[21] So your "cardio" and overall metabolic health is well looked after with short bursts of high effort/high energy output muscular activity—whether you choose to use only your bodyweight (as in running and calisthenics) or resistance (such as strength training) really makes no difference at all to your body, so long as its muscles are worked in such a manner that all classes of skeletal muscle fibers are thoroughly activated.

CARDIO & FAT LOSS

This being said, the reality is that most people who pose the question "what about my cardio?" couldn't care less about their blood vessels, arteries, or the health of their hearts. They're way more interested in losing body fat and have been told that cardio equals aerobic, and aerobic equals fat burning. This is simply a misconception built upon a false assumption.

To be sure, there is no such thing as a "fat loss exercise." Any fat that you see is simply a sign that a surplus of energy has been consumed. And any energy consumed beyond that which the body requires to fuel its vital life processes and activity levels is simply stored in your body in the form of fat cells.

All exercise first draws energy from a limited supply that exists within the muscles in the form of adenosine triphosphate, or ATP. When this supply runs out the body will utilize whatever glycogen is stored in the particular set of muscles that are being trained. When the glycogen supply runs down, the body will start to manufacture more glycogen through a process that takes place in the liver known as gluconeogenesis. If the muscular activity that you are engaging in is carried on beyond this point, oxygen will be required and the preferred fuel will be fatty acids. Once this happens, you can continue your activity (assuming the pace isn't too demanding) for a long period of time. A pound of fat, for example, contains a lot of energy—somewhere between 3,500 and 4,423.90[22] calories. However, if you were looking to burn a pound of fat from running, it might help you to know that running a mile will burn (depending upon your weight) approximately 100 calories. Do the math: Are you prepared to carry on your running activity nonstop for 35 to 44 miles in order to lose one pound of fat? And even if you are that dedicated, the amount of fat you will end up losing through such increased activity is much lower than you probably realize. A study published online in September 2009 in the *British Journal of Sports Medicine* reported that 58 obese people who completed 12 weeks of supervised aerobic ("cardio") training (which consisted of five cardio workouts per week) lost an average of a little more than seven pounds, with the majority losing less than half that amount.[23] As you can see, low-intensity cardio activity simply doesn't burn that many calories. According to Dan Carey, PhD, an assistant professor of exercise physiology at the University of St. Thomas in Minnesota, who studies exercise and metabolism, "Walking, even at a very easy pace, you'll probably burn three or four calories a minute."[24] This is over and above what you might burn if you were sitting in a chair.

Without some sort of dietary reduction (calories, carbs, fats, proteins, etc.) fat loss from exercise alone is at best an exercise in futility. Every client I've ever had who has decided to add, say, running to a reduced-calorie diet in order to lose fat has ended up with a diet that isn't so calorie reduced, as the body sends very strong biological prompts to replenish the energy that was output during one's daily runs. In fact, an interesting study by Harvard University was reported in the *Daily Mail*[25] in which the results of 64 individuals who were put on a marathon running training program in an effort to lose weight were analyzed. The results showed that 78 percent of those involved didn't lose any weight at all. Only 11 percent lost any weight, and this was washed out by the fact that the remaining 11 percent gained weight. And of those that gained weight, almost all of them were women. The study reported that three quarters of the women in the study reported eating more food. You've heard the phrase "working up an appetite"? Well that's exactly what happens when you output a steady stream of energy on a frequent basis; your body wants it back—with interest. Do this several days a week and pretty soon your body's demand for inputting energy back into the system will quickly outweigh the mind's willingness to restrict energy input.

The ultra-thin athletes that you see gracing the pages of running magazines had a genetic predisposition for being thin long before they began running. In other words, they were thin *prior to* their running, not *because of* it. Such a body type (ultra-thin) is the ideal body type for successful running, particularly running marathons, since less body mass has to be transported (less muscular work, less energy output) over the distance and the duration of the run.

Since the activity of running burns so few calories, one has to wonder how it somehow became associated in so many people's minds with fat loss. Again, it certainly couldn't be the calorie-burning component of the activity—unless you're running so often and for so long that you simply don't have time or opportunity to eat, which is rather a convoluted way to avoid putting food in your mouth (and more a testament to one's lack of self-control than it is to the diligence paid to one's exercise program).

Most personal trainers of any experience know that a six-pack is made in the kitchen—not in the gymnasium or on the running track. This became evident to me during an informal study that we conducted some years back, wherein 33 clients were put through a 10-week diet and strength-training program that saw them eat a balanced but calorie-reduced diet. Every two weeks their energy intake was reduced by 100 calories until the men were only consuming 1,300 and the women 1,000 calories a day for the final two weeks of the study. The subjects had been training for a year prior to starting the study and their ages ranged from 20 to 65. Prior to the study their body composition was tested and it was continuously tested every two weeks once the study started. The subjects started off with a workout consisting of one set each of six different exercises and trained but once a week. After two weeks their number of exercises was cut back from six to four, and the subjects' body composition was tested to see how they were progressing. For the first five weeks of the study whenever the subjects were tested it was discovered that not only had they lost fat, but they had also lost muscle, which had not been expected or desired. In an effort to correct this, the subjects' workout volume was cut back to one set each of three exercises and when their composition was tested again it was noted that they didn't lose any more muscle, but they did lose more fat. So, to test a hypothesis, the group was then divided in two, with half of them sticking with the three-exercise workout once a week, and the other half performing a two-exercise workout once a week. And to our surprise, when the data was examined at the end of the study, the group that had reduced the volume of their workouts to one set of two exercises and trained but once a week gained twice as much muscle and lost twice as much fat than did any other group. Indeed, when the data at the end of the 10-week study was examined more critically, it was discovered that a workout consisting of two sets once a week outperformed a three-set workout, a four-set workout, and a six-set workout—despite the subjects being at their lowest calorie intake during the entire program.

What this study revealed was the fact that when calories are restricted in a fat loss program (which they need to be if fat loss is the goal), a two-minute exercise program contributed more to the fat loss process than did exercise programs of longer duration. Again, the reality is that exercise doesn't burn that many calories, and doing as much exercise as you can tolerate (as in the case of the marathoners) can actually cause you to gain weight, as it will spike your appetite dramatically. Further, losing body fat can be a very stressful process to your body, resulting in stress hormones making an impact on your physiology and metabolism. Just the act of reducing your daily energy intake is stressful to the body. And when the body is under stress, burdening it with a frequent stress-producing activity (such as exercise) may result in the body becoming reluctant to let go of its stored energy (body fat), as with all of this energy going out and very little coming in, the body perceives that it is in a low energy-yielding environment that is threatful to its survival. Consequently, fat (which is stored energy after all) becomes a very desirable thing to have around.

In conclusion, one doesn't require daily cardio sessions in order to lose body fat. It's not that such activities don't burn calories—they do, and, if calorie intake is closely regulated, such activities can contribute to burning some body fat—but they just burn so few calories that they're not really worth engaging in, particularly given the high wear and tear factor of most cardio exercises. I do believe that it is important that one remain active, however, as this sends the appropriate metabolic message to the brain that all is well and that carrying stored body fat is not necessary as you are quite capable of moving and, thus, locating energy (food). However, it isn't necessary to have a regimented cardio session performed at a modest level of intensity for it to be that way. All that's required is for one to be *normally* active.

One must keep in mind that every time one outputs energy—however low the intensity—one is going to receive a strong biological prompt to input energy back into the system again. And if one outputs energy on a daily basis that is at a level that is higher than normal, it's going to take a will of iron to resist those constant internal signals telling you to replace the energy that you've used up through activity. This is precisely why the sales of "cardio" machines, such as treadmills, have never been higher, and yet our national levels of obesity have also never been higher.

CHAPTER SIX

YOGA FOR HEALTH AND STRETCHING FOR FLEXIBILITY

I f activities such as running contribute little to the fat-loss process, there is another popular activity that contributes even less, despite the fact that an entire industry has grown up around it. And this activity is yoga.

Some of my clients believe that yoga is a good supplemental activity to perform that will help them to achieve better health and lose body fat. Unfortunately, there is little scientific evidence for either belief, which mostly originates from crafty marketing. With regard to losing body fat, a study conducted in 2006 discovered that the long-term practice of yoga actually reduced the practitioner's resting metabolic rate, thus slowing the rate at which their bodies burned calories. This was particularly true for the women in the study.[1]

With regard to the claims regarding yoga's healing and health-promoting capabilities, these would appear to have been grossly overstated. In November 2015 the Australian government's Department of Health conducted an extensive review of yoga's alleged therapeutic effect (in addition to examining 16 other alternative healing therapies that were covered by private insurance) and could not conclude that yoga delivered *any* meaningful results.[2] The objective of the review was to summarize the evidence for the effectiveness and, where available, the safety, quality, or cost-effectiveness of yoga for a variety of clinical conditions. The reviewers looked at any systematic reviews that had been published since 2008 that focused on the use of yoga for the management of any clinical condition in terms of health outcomes. They analyzed 67 studies, including:

- 19 trials that treated arthritis and musculoskeletal conditions (such as carpal tunnel syndrome, fibromyalgia syndrome, kyphosis, low back pain, osteoarthritis, and rheumatoid arthritis.
- 15 trials that treated cancer
- 11 trials that treated cardiovascular disease
- 1 trial that treated insomnia
- 6 trials that dealt with yoga's effects on menopause
- 25 trials that examined yoga's effect on mental health conditions
- 5 trials that improved cognitive function
- 4 trials that dealt with yoga's effect on health problems in pediatric patients, including attention deficit hyperactivity disorder
- 4 trials that examined yoga's effect on pregnancy and labor
- 1 trial on yoga's effect on renal disease
- 14 trials dealing with the treatment of respiratory conditions with yoga
- 2 trials examining yoga's impact on smoking cessation
- 6 trials dealing with yoga's effects on type 2 diabetes/metabolic syndrome

After all of this analysis, the conclusion of the reviewers was:

> There is weak evidence that yoga improves symptoms in people with depression compared with control (i.e., those who did not practice yoga). For all other clinical conditions in which yoga was assessed there was insufficient evidence to draw any conclusions about the effect of yoga on outcomes.[3]

Although the evidence for yoga was far from conclusive with regard to its healing and health benefits, the evidence for its being an unsafe activity is mounting. A quick jog through the medical literature reveals that yoga practitioners have suffered all manner of problems—fatal air embolisms have been noted after engaging in yoga's breathing exercises[4]; hip damage can occur (particularly in women between the ages of 30 and 40)[5]; Femoroacetabular Impingement (F.A.I.), a condition caused by damaged cartilage, inflammation, pain, and arthritis, was reported in the *New York Times*[6] and, according to the author of the *Times* piece,

William Broad, "I found that hundreds of orthopedic surgeons in the Mediterranean region heard a conferred presentation in 2010 that linked F.A.I. to middle-aged women who do yoga."[7]

Then there is the case of elderly women, or those with conditions such as osteopenia or osteoporosis, who are seeking to become healthy and fit but who must also be very careful of what exercises they can do so as not to risk damaging their bones. As movements involving spinal flexion are not uncommon in yoga, it shouldn't really surprise us to learn of the results of a study from Mehrsheed Sinaki, MD, of the Mayo Clinic involving three women, aged 61, 70, and 87, who were diagnosed with osteopenia but who were otherwise healthy, that developed spinal fractures as a result of taking yoga.[8] If you are unhealthy presently but are thinking of taking yoga as a gentle means of regaining your health, you should know that when a large-scale survey of 2,508 yoga practitioners in Japan was completed it revealed that 30 percent of yoga class attendees had experienced some type of adverse event.[9]

In another article published in the *New York Times* by the same William Broad entitled "How Yoga Can Wreck Your Body," it was revealed that trapped nerves, stretched ligaments, and even strokes (among a host of other ailments) can be very real threats to the average yoga practitioner. According to Broad:

> . . . a growing body of medical evidence supports [40-year yoga instructor Glenn] Black's contention that, for many people, a number of commonly taught yoga poses are inherently risky. The first reports of yoga injuries appeared decades ago, published in some of the world's most respected journals—among them, *Neurology*, *The British Medical Journal* and *The Journal of the American Medical Association*. The problems ranged from relatively mild injuries to permanent disabilities.[10]

Some yoga devotees might argue that of course certain postures in yoga might be dangerous, but if you avoid those postures you can perform the activity without threat of injury. The problem, however, is how does a beginner to the discipline determine which postures are going to be dangerous for him or her *a priori*?

A NOT-SO-ANCIENT DISCIPLINE

There exists an unfounded belief that the yoga we see practiced today is thousands of years old and has been passed down from generation to generation, and, consequently, any potentially harmful elements in it have been filtered out as the discipline was passed down over the generations. The belief is that only the good stuff (i.e., the safe and gentle elements) has been passed down over the millenniums until it ultimately found its way to your local yoga class. The reality, however, is that yoga enjoys no such antiquity.

The yoga we see practiced today is about as old as the author of this book. Indeed, many of the postures within yoga are late add-ons to the discipline. The route to modern yoga began approximately 200 years ago when an Indian Prince (Krishnaraja Wodeyar III) produced a manual called "Sritattvanidhi" which featured about 122 poses taken primarily from gymnastics, rather than from ancient spiritual texts. In 1960 B. K. S. Lyengar combined certain of these poses with certain Hindu texts and—voila!—yoga, as we know it, was born. In other words what many people believe to be a highly spiritual discipline that is thousands of years old is in reality—as stated by author C. Covile in his article at cracked.com—"a chanted-up version of an early 20th-century gym class."[11]

For those into history, the oldest authentic yoga literature indicating what postures are to be performed can be found in the *Yoga Pradipika*, which was authored in the fifteenth century, and revealed a mere 32 poses, half of which were performed seated and did not include any of the push-ups, sun salutations, inversions, downward dog, or revolved triangle postures that we see today. So, yes, if the bulk of the yoga you intend to do will be performed from a motionless sitting position, then you will probably be quite safe. However, such a posture isn't that different from one assumed by a couch potato, and nobody would claim any spiritual, exercise, or health benefit from that posture.

STRETCHING TO PREVENT INJURY

One of the beliefs advanced in favor of activities such as yoga is that the stretching exercises that are part of the discipline will serve to make the practitioner far more limber and flexible, and thus reduce the chances that the practitioner will incur an injury. And while stretching is common in yoga, it is not exclusive to that discipline. Athletes in almost every sport routinely perform stretching as an activity unto itself. In my hometown of Bracebridge, Ontario, the most popular local team sport is hockey, which, like most sports, has more than its share of ritualism. It is not uncommon to see players skate to their respective ends of the rink prior to the start of a game and begin a very elaborate stretching ritual that is intended to warm up the players' muscles, ligaments, and tendons. It is believed that by the performance of this activity the players will become more supple and their muscles more pliable, thereby enhancing their preparedness to play and simultaneously reducing their chance of injury in what is a fast and often violent game.

Certain studies on injuries in athletics have concluded that "most organized sports-related injuries (60 percent) occur during practice,"[12] and, of course, chief among the warm-up rituals in most organized sports practices is stretching. And while athletes continue to stretch in order to reduce their chances of injury, scientists are issuing reports and results of studies that are calling the practice of stretching for this purpose into serious question. Indeed, a report issued by the Centers for Disease Control and Prevention (CDC) and published in the American College of Sports Medicine journal, *Medicine and Science in Sports and Exercise*, concluded rather categorically that stretching does *not* reduce the chance of injury.[13] Stephen B. Thacker, the director of the epidemiology program at the CDC, along with four colleagues, combed through the research databases for studies that compared stretching with other ways thought to prevent training injuries. They actually combined data from five studies in order to look more thoroughly for any benefits that might come to light as a pattern. After such a lengthy analysis they concluded that people who stretch were *not* less likely to suffer injuries (such as pulled muscles), and that stretching in and of itself did nothing to prevent injuries from occurring. Even more startling were the conclusions of an earlier study[14] of Honolulu Marathon runners that concluded that stretching prior to exercise was more likely to cause injury than to prevent it. The study, conducted by David A. Lally, PhD, an exercise physiologist at the University of Hawaii-Manoa, analyzed 1,543 individuals who participated in the Honolulu Marathon, and his key finding—that stretching was associated with more injuries—would certainly come as a shock to a lot of coaches if they would trouble themselves to read the science literature, as opposed to merely adopting the pre-game warm-up rituals of professional sports teams.

Additional science articles have been published that have reviewed hundreds of studies on stretching, and all of these have come to essentially the same conclusion: that stretching before an activity does not help to prevent injury.[15] One study conducted by the Physiotherapy Department at Kapooka Health Centre in New South Wales, Australia, investigated the effect of muscle stretching performed as a warm-up on the risk of exercise-related injury. They were able to oversee a huge database of 1,538 male army recruits who were randomly allocated to either a stretching or a control group. During the ensuing 12 weeks of training both groups performed active warm-up exercises before their physical training sessions, with the stretching group performing the additional warm-up of one 20-second static stretch under supervision for each of six major leg muscle groups. This was done during every warm-up session. The control group did not stretch. The researchers concluded that "a typical muscle stretching protocol performed during pre-exercise as a warm-up does not produce clinically meaningful reductions in risk of exercise-related injury."[16]

STRETCHING AS WARM-UP

During an interview on Canadian radio (C.B.C's Radio One in Vancouver, B.C.), researcher Paul Ingraham said that the idea of warming up a muscle by stretching it was akin to "trying to cook a steak by pulling on it." According to Ingraham:

> Body heat is generated by *metabolic activity*, particularly muscle contractions. The best way to warm up is to start doing a kinder, gentler version of the activity you have in mind: walk before you run. You simply cannot warm up your muscles by stretching them.[17]

Moreover, if one stretches one's muscles before they have been warmed up it can actually increase one's chance of injury. Taking a "cold" muscle and putting it in the weakest position in its range of motion (i.e., the fully stretched position) and then applying force to it (either the weight of the body or through the application of muscular force) is a very direct way to injure muscles and connective tissues.

STRETCHING & FLEXIBILITY

Over the decades the research into the alleged benefits of stretching has revealed some additional surprises, most notably that stretching doesn't increase an athlete's flexibility and, indeed, can serve to actually *reduce* an athlete's flexibility. In a study published in the *British Journal of Sports Medicine*, the researchers concluded that, "the flexibility index decreased significantly after stretching training."[18] It must be remembered that muscles have a fixed range over which they can be moved and this is as it must be in order for the muscles, and the joints that serve them, to be protected. You can only stretch as far as your muscles, tendons, and ligaments will allow you—and attempting to stretch beyond such limitations can be dangerous, as it can result in a weakening of the tendons and ligaments.

Quite apart from its inert or decidedly negative effects, stretching to enhance one's flexibility may, in the long run, be a delusion. According to Dr. Malachy McHugh, the director of research for the Nicholas Institute of Sports Medicine and Athletic Trauma at Lenox Hill Hospital in New York, being extremely flexible may not be desirable and is extremely limited by one's genetics. Only a small percentage of each person's flexibility is adaptable, says McHugh, "but it takes a long time and a lot of work to get even that small adaptation. It's depressing, really. . . . You only see changes in the actual, physical structure of the muscles after months of stretching for hours at a time. Most people aren't going to do that."[19] And finally the good doctor declares:

> Flexibility is a functional thing. You only need enough range of motion in your joints to avoid injury. More is not necessarily better.[20]

STRETCHING & STRENGTH

Strength is obviously important in athletics, as that attribute allows an individual to perform with greater speed and power, and also protects him from injury by fortifying the structures that support his bones and joints. In an attempt to increase strength, athletes and their trainers have engaged in many different approaches to tax an athlete's musculature, ranging from having them contract their muscles against various resistance apparatus such as rubber bands and barbells. More recently, stretching has been put forth as an activity that can serve to strengthen muscle tissue, with the result that many athletes now engage in stretching with the belief that their doing so will serve to make them stronger. However, a study presented at the 2006 meeting of the American College of Sports Medicine (ACSM) looked into what actual effect stretching had on the development of strength, and its conclusions did not lend support to the proposition that stretching is a viable means of strengthening muscle tissue.

The study featured 18 college students who performed a one-rep-maximum test of knee flexion after doing either: zero, one, two, three, four, five, or six 30-second hamstring stretches. The experimenters discovered that performing just one 30-second stretch significantly reduced (rather than increased) strength in the athletes' one-rep maximum performances by 5.4 percent. After the subjects performed six 30-second stretches, their strength *declined* by 12.4 percent.[21] The conclusion the ACSM reached is that stretching—even for as little as 30 seconds—makes one weaker, not stronger. Since no athlete wants to be weaker and more susceptible to injury, stretching is not something that any serious athlete should engage in, particularly just prior to a game or competition. According to Ingraham, simply performing the type of activity that they will be required to do in competition but doing so at a kinder, gentler pace—e.g., a light skate, such as hockey players often do, prior to the start of the game, will cause the muscles the athletes will be using to contract, which will draw blood into those same muscles, making them more pliable and, thus, less prone to sudden strain. There is also evidence that the act of stretching interferes with one's neural control of muscles, leading to a weaker contraction. A different experiment that looked into this issue found a 28 percent reduction in maximum voluntary muscle contraction, which remained depressed by 9 percent for a full hour after the stretching ended.[22] In plain English, stretching produced a weaker muscle contraction. Furthermore, researchers at Florida State conducted a study that revealed that trained distance runners who stretched before they ran became 5 percent less efficient and covered 3 percent less distance in a time trial. This revealed not only the immediate weakening of muscle as a result of stretching but also how static stretching negatively impacted endurance performance.[23]

In conclusion, stretching really doesn't do any of the things (from warming up, to preventing injuries, to strengthening, to staving off soreness, to enhancing flexibility) that the old paradigm previously assumed that it did, but it does do something that most trainers and coaches didn't anticipate—it makes you weaker. So the ritual of having athletes engage in stretching before their practices and games will send them into an important athletic competition weaker and, thus, more prone to being injured, inadequately warmed up, and not able to generate the power that they might need to produce a sudden burst of speed in order to make a play, get out of harm's way, take a more powerful shot, kick a ball harder, and sprint faster down a field. Instead, the performance of stretching simply results in the athlete performing on a subpar level.

CHAPTER SEVEN

ATHLETICS FOR FITNESS

When the realization dawns on many of us that we need to get back in shape, many will consider a return to certain sports that we performed when we were younger and fitter. You might have been a pretty decent figure skater, baseball, or hockey player back in the day and you were in pretty good shape then, if you recall correctly, so why not join a recreational league? Or play some pickup basketball? Besides, look at the condition of the professional athletes that play these sports—great endurance, lithe grace, and very low levels of body fat. Hell, who wouldn't want to look at least a little more like one of these guys?

Indeed. It's little wonder that many of us look at these exceptional athletes as being prime examples of physical fitness and health—and why wouldn't we? Well, perhaps because what we are really seeing when we look at such individuals are members of our species who were born with a genetic predisposition to excel at certain physical activities and who, through thousands of hours of practice, have become extraordinarily proficient at skill sets that are specific to the sport they play. What we're *not* seeing is the long-term damage that all of the rigorous athletic training and competition is doing to the bodies of these same individuals. Indeed, a survey that was conducted with 15,000 athletes from the University of Alabama's alumni department did just that, examining the effect that competing in varsity level athletics had on the health and fitness levels of the athletes who participated in them. The authors of this survey concluded that:

The price many athletes pay to compete is high. Based on these data, some athletes sacrifice their future quality-of-life for their athletic participation in youth athletics, high school, and collegiate sport. Sports are an important part of American culture, but the long-term risks are rarely considered. Increased risk of disability, obesity, and chronic disease may be what a competitive athlete . . . will face.[1]

In young athletes (aged five to 14), who are among the most active athletically, the injury rate is equally as shocking. According to the Children's Hospital Boston (the primary pediatric teaching hospital of Harvard Medical School), of the approximately 30 million children and teens who participate in some form of organized sports each year, three million of them (or 10 percent) will end up hurt as a result. Indeed, the data indicates that one-third of all injuries suffered during childhood will be caused by their participation in sports.[2]

According to statistics amassed by the National SAFE KIDS Campaign and the American Academy of Pediatrics (AAP):

1. Sports and recreational activities contribute to approximately 21 percent of all traumatic brain injuries among American children and adolescents.
2. More than 775,000 children and adolescents ages 14 and under are treated in hospital emergency rooms for sports-related injuries each year. Most of the injuries occur as a result of falls, being struck by an object, collisions, and overexertion during unorganized or informal sports activities.
3. More severe injuries occur during individual sports and recreational activities.
4. Most organized sports-related injuries (60 percent) occur during practice.
5. Approximately 20 percent of children and adolescents participating in sports activities are injured each year, and one in four injuries is considered serious.
6. Sports-related injury severity increases with age.

7. Overuse injury, which occurs over time from repeated motion, is responsible for nearly half of all sports injuries to middle and high school students. Immature bones, insufficient rest after an injury, and poor training or conditioning contribute to overuse injuries among children.

INJURIES ON A PER SPORT BASIS

Given the amount of money that changes hands at the professional level of organized sports, you don't see a lot of major sponsors of professional sports teams investing in scientific studies on safety. Consequently, one has to go back a few years to find studies that reveal the number of injuries incurred on a per sport basis. The following represents a sample taken just in the United States in 1998, indicating the number of children (aged five to 14) who were injured seriously enough to require hospital emergency room treatment, and the various sports that caused these injuries:

1. Basketball – 200,000
2. Baseball – 91,000
3. Softball – 26,000 (incidentally, baseball also had the highest fatality rate among sports for children aged five to 14, with three to four children dying from baseball injuries each year)
4. Bicycling – 320,000 (in addition, 225 children died in bicycle-related accidents in 1997)
5. Football – 159,000
6. Gymnastics – 25,500
7. Ice Hockey – 18,000 (statistics from 2001–2002)
8. Ice Skating – 10,600
9. In-line skating and/or rollerblading – 27,200
10. Skateboarding – 27,500
11. Sledding – 8,500
12. Snow skiing – 13,500
13. Snow boarding – 9,000
14. Soccer – 77,500
15. Trampoline – 80,000[3]

In other words, if you select athletics as your preferred method of exercise, there's a very big risk involved, and you will probably be injured either during training or in competition. Or, like the varsity athletes cited earlier, you could well end up with an "increased risk of disability, obesity and chronic disease."

Granted, athletes do develop great motor skills for the specific sport in which they compete, but what that has to do with health, fitness, or longevity has never been established. What has been established, however, is that participating in sports takes a large toll on health—with very few exceptions. In a study conducted by Brian P. Hamill, various sports that were performed within the United Kingdom and the United States were examined and then evaluated based on the amount of injuries incurred per 100 hours of participation by the athletes.[4] He summarized his findings as follows:

MULTI-SPORT COMPARATIVE INJURY RATES

SPORT	INJURIES PER 100 PARTICIPATION HOURS
Schoolchild soccer	-- 6.20
UK rugby	-- 1.92
South African rugby	-- 0.70
UK basketball	-- 1.03
USA basketball	-- 0.03
UK cross-country	-- 0.37
USA cross-country	-- 0.00
Fives	-- 0.21
P.E.	-- 0.18
Squash	-- 0.10
USA football	-- 0.10
Badminton	-- 0.05
USA gymnastics	-- 0.044
UK tennis	-- 0.07
USA powerlifting	-- 0.0027

USA tennis	-- 0.001
Rackets	-- 0.03
USA volleyball	-- 0.0013
Weight training	-- 0.0035 (85,733 hrs)
Weightlifting	0.0017 (168,551 hrs)[5]

In considering the above figures, it should be pointed out that these represent merely those injuries that required hospital emergency room attention—these do not include injuries that were incurred but did not require hospitalization (such as strains, cuts, bruises, etc.). If it did, then their inclusion would have increased these numbers considerably. Imagine for a moment what would happen if rather than sports events, the above statistics represented the injury rate incurred from jobs or classes in secondary schools. Would you, for instance, be comfortable sending your child into a class knowing that 10 percent of its students would be hurt to the point of requiring emergency room hospitalization or that their attending such classes would result in an "increased risk of disability, obesity and chronic disease?" One would hope not. Indeed, such a class would most likely be cancelled or at least boycotted until major steps were taken to remedy the situation. Nevertheless, when it comes to enrolling your child (or yourself) in sports it is (for some reason) believed by most that the health benefits to be had from engaging in such activities far outweigh the liabilities. Part of the reason for the high volume of injuries in sports is impact trauma. It's been calculated that jumping from even a height of 2.7 feet (80 centimeters) will result in a force of up to 20 times a person's body weight impacting one's ankles.[6] It doesn't take a statistician to figure out that doing this on a frequent basis can only lead to something bad happening eventually.

The reality is that there has never been (nor will there ever be) a link between sport and health, or sport and fitness. Everything from the battering athletes take during competition, to the damage caused by many of their practices (see point 4 above), to the often baseless and dangerous rituals passed along to them by various generations of coaches (such as stretching), to the influx of corporate dollars enticing them to embrace equipment, training programs, and nutritional practices that—at best—are ineffective, to the lure of ingesting powerful performance-enhancing drugs that can wreak havoc on one's arteries and glandular systems—all of these factors militate against athletics being a healthy pursuit or the best route to enhancing one's health and fitness.

When it comes to decisions about your health there are only two options, and they're not whether you are tough or timid, but whether you are smart or stupid. All in all, if you are looking to get back into shape and not cripple yourself in the process, you are best to look (particularly if you're outside of your teen years) elsewhere than athletic competition.

CHAPTER EIGHT

NUTRITIONAL SUPPLEMENTATION FOR SUPER HEALTH

It seems to be human nature to look for a path of least resistance in almost all walks of life. After all, who among us wouldn't like to achieve whatever it is that one so feverishly desires at a fraction of the going rate? And while this might be prudent from certain perspectives, I'm afraid such an attitude finds no purchase when it comes to exercise. Nevertheless, there exists a persistent belief within the health and fitness world that more or better results can be had if a magic bean of sorts could be added into the trainee's daily diet.

To wit, a client arrived at my training facility for his weekly appointment and, prior to his workout, we conversed about various things that were going on in our neighborhood. During the conversation he felt compelled to mention that a 24-hour gym had recently opened up, and that its manager was telling people about a special protein powder that he was selling through his facility that would make whomever took it "twice as strong" as they would be if they didn't take it. "If the protein powder could make one stronger all on its own, then what would be the necessity of the workout?" I asked. He nodded rather grimly in the affirmative, and then we headed into the training area of the gym. I put him through one of our typical high-energy output workouts, wherein he trained each exercise hard enough to ensure that he had tapped all three classes of muscle fibers in all of his major muscle groups. Upon completion of the workout he found that he needed to sit down to catch his breath and to allow his energy reserves a little more time than usual to recover and replenish before he headed home. During this time I juxtaposed what he had told me about the alleged properties of the protein supplement with the workout he had just completed. During the workout he had output a tremendous amount of energy—and he had done this for a reason; i.e., he knew that he had to empty the gas tanks in his muscles as thoroughly as possible in order to prompt his body to produce the positive change of building bigger, stronger muscles (in other words, to build him a "bigger gas tank," to continue with the metaphor).

The client understood that he had engaged in a stimulus-response relationship that was predicated on high-energy output. Such workouts are not easy; they go against the grain of everything that the body "likes" to experience, but outputting such large amounts of energy is the reason why his body would then be prompted to make the adaptive change that it would. High-energy output is the stimulus the body requires in order to be prompted to invest in positive biological change. It has to be high-energy output; even low-to-moderate energy output doesn't cut it. This being the case, I asked him how consuming a powder (which is an example of energy *input*) could act to facilitate a transformation that is solely a response to an energy-*output* stimulus? He acknowledged my point—that there was no high-energy-output taking place when inputting energy—and yet we both understood that the protein powder he had told me about would continue to be sold to unsuspecting clients at the neighborhood gym (and perhaps in other gyms throughout North America as well) as being a stimulus for muscle growth. And the reason why this is, and why such supplements will always have a market, is our species' deeply ingrained desire to get more of what we want with less effort than would normally be required. Given that it soon becomes evident to trainees that a large effort is required in order to cause one's body to produce any positive result at all, it doesn't take long before most people begin looking outside of the workout itself to the world of nutritional supplementation to see if certain of its products might just produce a better return on one's energy investments at the gym. With no shortage of products to sell, and an almost built-in human predilection to seek out such products, the nutritional supplement industry has been exploiting this natural impulse in humans for as long as commerce has intersected human concerns regarding their health and fitness.

While I have decried the snake oil nature of the supplement industry in my previous books, the supplement industry nevertheless endures. Indeed, it has grown. I know that I would be a considerably wealthier man today if I created my own brand of supplements to sell out of my facility and through my social media outlets to a steady stream of clients who look to me for guidance and science-based advice. I just can't do it. When I first opened my facility a man that I used to work with when I was a sports reporter for a local newspaper showed up to tell me of a wonderful supplement he was now selling that was an "energy extender." When a former colleague begins lying to you in order to make a buck it's sad. Nevertheless, he extolled its virtues: "It extends your energy but has no calories." When I told my wife, Terri, this, she responded, "Wow. It has energy but no calories? What's it made of—air?" After all, "energy drinks" are able to be called energy drinks because they contain calories—that is to say, *energy*—and not because they make you more energetic by consuming them. When I expressed my skepticism the man snorted, "It's been tested scientifically!"—hoping that his declaration would suffice to put the matter to rest and get me on board to carry the product. "Bring me the science studies that have been done on it and I'll consider it," I said. The man promised he would return with the studies and left. That was 12 years ago and I haven't seen him since.

Several years later a woman came to my facility to inquire about signing up for my workout services.

"I want to get stronger and rebuild some muscle that I've lost," she began. "But before I sign up I should tell you that I own the new herbal diet company that just opened up in town."

After a pause to ensure that she had my attention she continued.

"Now I've heard about your opinion of supplements from other people in town and I don't know that I can be supporting you by buying a membership at your facility if you're not supporting me."

Fair enough, I thought. I told her that I had never seen any evidence that supplements did what their manufacturers and marketers suggested and that I had direct experience with the problems of herbal supplements in particular (a personal trainer once gave me a multi-vitamin that contained ephedrine, which sent my heart off like a trip hammer) and also there had been some serious health problems attributed to certain herbal concoctions (remember, the supplement industry is unregulated, meaning that all sorts of things can go into a supplement without first testing what the long-term effects on people's health will be). Long story short: she decided not to join my facility. Later on, another client of mine brought in some advertising materials from the woman's weight-loss facility. I was struck by one line in her advertisement that stated that by taking her supplements one would "build lean tissue" (i.e., muscle). If that were truly the case, why then would she have sought out my services in the first place? If she honestly believed that the herbal supplement she was selling would stimulate her body to build muscle in and of itself she would never have felt the need to seek out my services, as she could have obtained whatever results my facility could provide solely from the ingestion of her herbal pills. It was another case of appealing to people's desire to get something without having to expend the energy necessary to acquire it.

SUPPLEMENTS & HEALTH

I find it contemptible that people with no interest in the health and well-being of their clients enter the health and fitness industry with the assumption that everyone in it is a sucker to be taken advantage of. But, alas, some people do. And every year more and more people willingly yield to their bodies' innate desire to conserve energy and their mind's desire to achieve the appearance of bodies that have output a lot of energy to appear the way they do. Unfortunately for them, nutritional supplements have, at best, been shown to be inert, but, at worst, they can actually do a body more harm than good. Witness, for example, a study that followed 38,772 older women who frequently used supplements for a period of 25 years, which revealed that their risk of death *increased* with their long-term use of the supplements B6, iron, magnesium, folic acid, copper, and multi-vitamins, causing the authors of the study to conclude that there exists, "little justification for the general and widespread use of dietary supplements."[1]

Another study, this one examining 35,533 men over a 10-year period, examined whether the supplements vitamin E and/or selenium would help to reduce the risk of colon cancer in this population. The researchers split the subjects into four groups, each receiving daily supplementation of vitamin E only, selenium only, vitamin E and selenium together, or nothing at all (in the form of placebo tablets). At the end of the study the researchers discovered that the subjects' risk of cancer *increased* for the men who took the supplements (either vitamin E and selenium together or taking them individually). While the increased risk was small, it was enough to establish that by taking the supplements the men were heading in the opposite direction of successfully staving off prostate cancer.[2]

VITAMIN C

Many people who grew up in my generation might well be tempted to excuse vitamin C from this chapter. I know that my mother, who was a registered nurse by training, often insisted that her children had a vitamin C supplement present with at least one of our meals or, if shopping for a multi-vitamin, she ensured that it would contain an extra measure of this particular vitamin. And she was not the only mother who brought ascorbic acid into the home for family consumption. When the chemist and Nobel Laureate Linus Pauling published his book in 1970 declaring that mega-doses of this vitamin actually prevented the common cold, innumerable families immediately purchased high-dose supplemental vitamin C and took several of these tablets daily. After all, a Nobel Laureate certainly must know what he is talking about, mustn't he? After the passing of several decades of research into the matter, it is not entirely clear that he did. A review conducted in 2005 that covered 50 years' worth of research on the subject concluded that, "the lack of effect [of vitamin C curing the common cold] . . . throws doubt on the utility of this wide practice."[3] Indeed. And while vitamin C was not shown to prevent the common cold, it was revealed that such high doses of it did in fact increase one's risk of developing kidney stones and severe diarrhea.[4]

VITAMIN A AND BETA CAROTENE

The vitamins C, A, and E have been classified as antioxidants, which are believed to help fight diseases such as cancer. The evidence, however, doesn't support this. In a large study supported by the National Cancer Institute, smokers who consumed vitamin A were more likely to get lung cancer than those who did not.[5] The vitamin A advocates like to point out that the vitamin serves to keep your eyes and skin healthy, but they seldom mention that having too much of it can actually be toxic, producing multiple side effects such as bleeding in the lungs, blurry vision, bone pain, breathing difficulty, changes in immune function, chronic inflammation of the liver, cirrhosis (scarring of the liver), cough, cracked fingernails, cracked lips, decreased thyroid function, depression, diarrhea, feeling of fullness, fever, fluid around the heart, hair loss, high cholesterol, increased pressure in the brain, increased risk of HIV transmission (through breastfeeding), increased risk of lung cancer, increased risk of heart disease, increased white blood cells, indigestion, inflammation of the conjunctiva (conjunctivitis), injection site pain, irritability, joint pain, mouth ulcers, muscle pain, psoriasis flare-ups, pain, perisinusoidal fibrosis (in the liver), redness (from skin use), respiratory infection, seizure, skin irritation, sore eyes, steatosis (fatty change), stomach and intestine adverse effectives, suicidal thoughts, and even death.[6]

THE B VITAMINS

Another group of vitamins that have come under closer scrutiny are the B vitamins, particularly B6 and B12. The National Institute of Health has indicated that taking B6 supplements for a long time can be more harmful than beneficial:

> People almost never get too much vitamin B6 from food. But taking high levels of vitamin B6 from supplements for a year or longer can cause severe nerve damage, leading people to lose control of their bodily movements.[7]

SPORTS SUPPLEMENTS VS. FAST FOOD

An even more startling revelation came as a result of a study comparing Sports Supplements, which are marketed as representing the cutting edge of scientific advancement in the areas of human recovery and peak performance, against common fast foods that you can pick up at any drive-through window. The result? No difference at all.[8] This study was conducted by a University of Montana graduate student named Michael Cramer, who tested to see if the claims of superiority from the multibillion dollar sports supplement industry were true. He compared the effect of supplements such as Gatorade, PowerBar, and Cytomas "energy powder" against the potency of burgers, fries, orange juice, hotcakes, and hash browns from a local McDonald's. For his subjects he selected 11 well-trained male athletes and, after having them fast 12 hours, they were made to partake in a rigorous 90-minute endurance workout. After the workout, the subjects were assigned to either a fast food group or a supplement group. The fast food group was given a hash brown, hotcakes, and orange juice, while the subjects assigned to the supplement group were given Cliff Shot Bloks, organic peanut butter, and Gatorade. Two hours later the fast food group were given a Coke, fries, and hamburger, while the supplement group were given Powerbar products and Cytomax powder. Two hours after this meal the subjects were then made to cycle over 12 miles on a stationary bike as quickly as they could. The calories and macronutrients of protein and carbohydrates were approximately equal in both groups, with slightly more sodium and fat being accounted for in the fast food group. The subjects then underwent blood work and muscle biopsies in order to determine their insulin, glycogen, lipid, and blood glucose levels. A week later the subjects were brought back into the lab and made to repeat their workouts, but this time they were assigned the diet opposite to the one they had been given the week before; i.e., the fast food group was given supplements and the supplement group was given fast food. After repeating the post workout testing, Cramer found that the performance of the athletes in cycling was just as fast after they ate fast food as it was after they consumed sports supplements. In other words, sports supplements did not provide a boost in performance ability, nor did they provide for faster recovery.

Nutritional supplements, it should be pointed out, were developed originally by medical researchers to provide just that—"supplementation"—to people who, through genetic or other gastrointestinal problems, were unable to either digest certain foods containing certain necessary vitamins and minerals or whose bodies were otherwise unable to extricate the necessary nutrients contained therein. They were never intended to be used by healthy individuals who were already consuming well-balanced diets, because medical and nutritional scientists understand that a healthy individual consuming a well-balanced diet is, by definition, getting everything he or she requires to be healthy from the foods he or she consumes—and the human body does not utilize nutrients beyond *need*. Despite the foregoing facts, many people continue to feel that they require more than their bodies require—and certainly more than a balanced diet would allot—of the various vitamins, minerals, and other nutrients. However, I can tell you categorically that this is simply not true.

THE PLACEBO EFFECT

A lot of the "success" that people report while taking a supplement comes solely from their belief that the supplement in fact does what it is advertised to do. When a trainee reads that a given athlete or celebrity took a certain supplement before he or she trained and that this resulted in he or she training harder and getting stronger, the trainee, believing himself to be similarly empowered by the supplement, will often train harder when taking it than he might have if he had not. But it is the harder training, rather than the supplement, that is the cause of his improved strength.

The placebo effect, or "power of suggestion," is really quite a remarkable phenomenon in and of itself, and has been observed in areas of human endeavor that lie far beyond supplement usage. The placebo effect in medicine, to indicate but one example, is not only well documented, but also startling in its magnitude. In one study that was conducted in Sweden, surgeons implanted pacemakers in 80 patients, but only turned on half (or 40) of them, leaving the other 40 pacemakers inactive. The inactive pacemakers were placebos, as the patients were not aware that they had not been turned on. However, after three months both groups of patients experienced improved heart function, while the placebo group was reported to have "significant improvement in perceived chest pain, dyspnea, and palpitations." The researchers concluded that the "pacemaker implantation had a placebo effect on objective and subjective parameters"[9] (i.e., the patients didn't just feel better; their hearts objectively performed better).

So how could an inert object implanted in one's chest result in such a positive effect taking place? Evidently it came down to the belief in the product by the patients, as the ones who received the "placebo" pacemaker honestly believed they were getting something that would help them. This, in combination with the fact that the patients' doctors told them that the pacemakers would help them, somehow brought about the physiological improvement that was noted. Again, the placebo effect is an amazing human capacity and offers at least one explanation as to why it is so difficult to test the effects of a drug or a food supplement, without knowing just how much the mind-set of the test subject influenced the results he or she might have experienced. This phenomenon can feed the manufacturer with hundreds or even thousands of earnest testimonial letters from customers who believe that the product they consumed actually worked. But there is one problem for the supplement manufacturers with all of this, and that is that the placebo effect has only been shown to work upon approximately 10 to 40 percent of people, resulting in the word of mouth promotion for a given product eventually fading away. Looked at mathematically, if only two people out of 10 who buy a product will feel inclined to recommend it to a friend, of those few new people only 20 percent will, in turn, recommend it to their friends, and so on. Consequently, the customer base grows smaller by the month, causing worried manufacturers to spend more on advertising (essentially throwing out a bigger net to catch a larger number of new customers). However, even this quickly reaches a point of diminishing returns and the board of directors within such companies quickly conclude that it is cheaper for them to announce an "all new" wonder supplement and start everyone off all over again than it is to keep beating what has clearly become a dead horse. This is why supplement companies are constantly bringing out new products. Very few of their products endure largely because the goal of super health is completely illusory. Health is merely the absence of disease; a body can either be healthy or unhealthy—and that's it. If you are deficient in a given nutrient then adding it into your diet either by food or by food supplement may bring you up to par—but no pill or powder is going to transcend this point and take you into the realm of super health.

Just remember that high-energy output is the stimulus for fat loss, as well as the production of cardiovascular health and strength. Supplements are an energy-in entity, and, barring the ability that certain of them possess to redress certain dietary imbalances owing to food allergies, they are (at best) inert. Well, that's not entirely true. They can also prompt your body to change the color of its urine as it attempts to process the surplus of a given nutrient out of one's system and, as we've seen, they can also further act to shorten one's life span.

CHAPTER NINE

BODYBUILDING FOR MASSIVE MUSCLES

Many young men and women have a natural desire to build up their bodies. Exceptional muscular development turns heads and gets one noticed. Among males, having larger than average size muscles can impart an aura of intimidation; i.e., if a well-built adversary presents himself, one knows that it will require more energy than perhaps one's own muscles possess to overpower or out-endure him. A larger muscle is a more powerful muscle and one that will typically function for longer periods of time than a smaller muscle, due to the fact that it has more energy (glycogen) stored inside of it. Consequently, the desire to have "bigger" muscles runs very high among males, particularly when in their prime years of 16 to 28, as those are the years in which they are most ready to compete for mates.

Taking advantage of this almost universal desire among young males, muscle magazines will typically enter into the picture and can easily lead these young men astray, as these magazines and their online counterparts are commercially driven entities whose sole existence is predicated on selling products, not on dispensing valid scientific training and nutritional advice. I recently clicked on a link sent to me by a client which took me to a page that revealed the arm routine of Arnold Schwarzenegger (aka the "Austrian Oak"). Now Schwarzenegger has been the poster boy for professional bodybuilding and supplement sales for over 40 years (since the mid 1970s) and he certainly did sport a freakishly large pair of arms. His biceps in particular were (and still are) something of a legend within the bodybuilding community, and so many young men desiring to increase the size of their arm muscles often try to follow the methods that Schwarzenegger employed. According to the online article:

. . . [Schwarzenegger] performed between 20 and 26 sets of [biceps] work twice a week, on Tuesday and Friday evenings.[1]

His actual biceps workout, according to the article, was as follows:

1. Cheating Barbell Curls: 5–8 sets for 8–12 repetitions each
2. Incline Dumbbell Curls: 5–8 sets for 8–12 repetitions each
3. One-arm Concentration Curls: 5 sets for 8–12 repetitions each
4. Standing Alternating Dumbbell Curls: 5 sets for 8–12 repetitions each

And this represents only the volume of exercise that Schwarzenegger performed for his biceps! According to the website bodybuildingology.com,[2] the "Austrian Oak" also dedicated a similar volume of exercise to target his triceps muscles (located on the back of the upper arms):

1. Close-Grip Bench Press: 5–6 sets of 6–8 repetitions
2. Cable Pressdowns: 5–6 sets of 6–8 repetitions
3. EZ-Bar French Presses: 5–6 sets of 6–8 repetitions
4. Dumbbell Kickbacks: 5 sets of 6–8 repetitions
5. Lying French Presses: 5 sets of 6–8 repetitions

Schwarzenegger's prescription, then, for building bigger arms was to perform 20 to 26 sets for biceps, and 25 to 28 sets for triceps, twice a week, for a weekly total of 90 to 108 sets of direct arm training. So, there you have it—the exercises, sets, and reps of "Bodybuilding's King of Kings" (this rather immodest moniker Schwarzenegger himself had coined and featured in one of his magazine ads to advertise his training courses back in the early 1980s). And, of course, since Schwarzenegger didn't just possess oversized arms, but also equally as prosperous muscles in his chest, back, shoulders, and legs, he recommended training the rest of one's muscle groups with a comparable amount of sets and repetitions over the course of a seven-day period. Indeed, such workouts were what Schwarzenegger claimed to have employed in training to win his various Mr. Olympia titles. All of this adds up to over 15 hours of time spent each week in the gym. From a practical standpoint, I don't know of anyone who has (or can afford) that kind of leisure time to devote to building up inordinately large muscles. More importantly, is that volume of resistance training really necessary in order for one to build bigger and stronger arms?

Interestingly, there was a study that explored just such a question. The study examined the results of two groups of resistance exercise trainees; the first group trained only with compound (multiple muscle groups involved simultaneously) movements such as Bench Presses, Lat Pulldowns, Dumbbell Incline Presses, and Dumbbell One-Arm Rows; the second group performed these same exercises but also added into their weekly training additional exercises for the biceps and triceps. According to the researchers:

> There were no significant differences between the groups in the percentage change before and after training. The findings of this study suggest that isolation exercises are not necessary in order to increase compound movement strength or increase upper-arm girth. These findings also suggest that strength coaches can save time by not including isolation exercises and still achieve increases in strength and size.[3]

In other words, if one's exercise program already contains exercises that involve the biceps and triceps muscles (such as Bench Presses, Pulldowns, Incline Presses, and Rows do), the addition of exercises that solely target the muscles of the upper arms is superfluous. You stimulated all of the upper arm musculature into growth that could be stimulated by performing the compound exercises. To therefore opt to spend more time exercising your arms when doing so will not result in any additional arm growth would appear to be time lost. As previously noted, time lost is time never to be recovered.

While the data would strongly suggest that "bodybuilding's king of kings" didn't need to perform nearly so much exercise as he did in order to develop his royal arms, it has to be said that a good portion of Mr. Schwarzenegger's physique was not the end result of his training methods. He had something when he started out on his bodybuilding training that the average person doesn't—exceptional genetics for building muscle. Indeed, photographs of Schwarzenegger taken when he was a teenager in Austria reveal a level of muscular development far beyond what most people could attain even after years of resistance training.

Similarly, I recall a conversation I had with the late Steve Reeves, the last of the great pre-steroid era bodybuilders and a man who carved out an incredibly successful film career for himself during the late 1950s and early 1960s largely (if not solely) as a result of his impressive physique. One afternoon at Reeves's ranch, Steve told me that he had been looking recently at some photographs of his late father, who died when Reeves was only 18 months old. "You know," Steve related, "my father had shoulders that were as broad as mine (Reeves was renowned for his shoulder-to-waist taper)—and yet my father never lifted a weight in his life."

As with all things that have a genetic component, there are reasons why the average person's muscle tissue typically exhibits a very limited growth capacity. First, if muscles were able to grow rapidly a person's movement potential would become compromised, as the angle of pull of a muscle across two joints would change dramatically (and not necessarily for the better). Second, a bigger muscle requires more energy to sustain it, which could be disastrous for a member of a species such as ours, which has struggled for centuries to pull enough energy (calories) out of its environment to survive. For this reason, a governor of sorts evolved into our genes to regulate the growth of our muscles. As Doug McGuff, MD, and I wrote in our book *Body By Science*:

A specific gene, which has been named GDF-8 (Growth and Differentiation Factor 8), produces a protein called Myostatin, the function of which is to stop differentiation of muscle stem cells or satellite cells from becoming larger. In other words, GDF-8 sets a ceiling on how large muscles can become. In most of us there is going to be a very generous expression of this GDF-8 gene, and therefore most of us will have a considerable amount of Myostatin circulating through our bodies, which, in turn, places a relatively modest level on how much muscle mass our bodies will produce.

Myostatin was first noted in Belgian cattle and while there is not much in the way of open plains in Belgium, nevertheless, the

Belgian cattle breeders were able to produce a type of bull that contained up to 30 percent more muscle mass than the average bovine. Evidently over a period of time and through selective breeding, they created this Herculean strain of bull which is now known as the Belgian Blue, the unique feature of which is that it carries two to three times the muscle mass of standard beef cattle (in the United States a similar process of selective breeding has resulted in a breed of cattle called the Peidmontese).

As more beef on the hoof results in greater meat yield (and hence greater money to be made) per head of cattle, researchers began to look into why the Belgian Blue was so freakishly large. To their surprise, they discovered that this strain of cattle was lacking a gene (GDF-8) that encoded for the Myostatin protein, and they believed that this was the source (or the cause) behind why these cattle had become so muscular.

Researchers Sejin Lee and Alexandra McPherron from Johns Hopkins University tested this theory by taking littermate mice (essentially twin mice) and subjecting them to a process that resulted in post-natal (or after birth) deletion of the GDF-8 gene and then they observed the response. In science, this method is known as Koch's Postulates (Koch's Postulates have to do with microbiology and disease, or how bacterium causes disease). Basically Koch's Postulates requires that if an animal has a disease, you isolate the suspected offending organism in a pure culture, then take that organism and inject it into a well animal. If that animal then gets the disease in question, then from that newly diseased animal you can again isolate the organism in pure culture. When you do this in a genetic sense, and you apply Koch's Postulates to myostatin, you take an animal that has the "disease" or condition in question—extremely massive muscles, in this instance—then you examine it, and find that it has a myostatin deletion. You then take an animal that is normal and produce a manipulation whereby its myostatin is deleted and that animal then becomes the abnormal animal with very large muscle mass. Then you set this as the master regulator for muscle growth (i.e., if this gene is deleted, then muscle mass increases). And that's the conclusion these researchers from Johns Hopkins came to; i.e., they were able to take GDF-8, which was presumed to be the cause of double muscling, and then they isolated it out from the animal and then—bang!—the mice they were testing became phenomenally over-muscled. This research confirmed that this gene and its lack of expression was the cause of the excess musculature.[4]

GENETICS DETERMINE RESPONSE

It's been estimated that if you were given a cross section of 100,000 adult males, perhaps only 20 would have the physical potential to grow muscles large enough to become champion bodybuilders. Thus, the odds for most young males to become massively muscled are very slight indeed. It simply isn't in the genetic cards for the vast majority of people to develop very large muscles. Apart from the role of myostatin indicated above, there are other genetic indices, such as IL-15RA, Ciliary Neurotrophic Factor (CNTF), Alpha-Actinin-3 (ACTN3), among others, and are estimated to account for 80 to 90 percent of the variations we see in muscle mass and strength among individuals.[5]

An interesting study indicating the supreme role of genetics in influencing one's response to bodybuilding exercise was conducted by Van Etten et al. In this study, two groups—one already muscular or mesomorphic, the other thin or ectomorphic—were each placed on an identical exercise program for 12 weeks and their results were closely monitored. At the completion of the study it was discovered that the mesomorphic group experienced significant gains in muscle mass, while the ectomorphic group experienced no significant improvement at all.[6] Therefore, those who are inordinately muscular to begin with will gain size and strength from their bodybuilding efforts to a much greater extent than those who are not naturally muscular or mesomorphic. Of course the bodybuilding industry ignores this, as it has long realized that the reality in such matters dramatically impedes commerce.

CLYDESDALES & MUSCLE MAGAZINES

Once one makes his/her peace with the fact that how big one's muscles ultimately can become is dependent upon one's genetic endowment, those that don't possess the necessary genetics to become massively muscled will, perhaps after an initial twinge of frustration, look at resistance training for the benefits it can actually impart and be happy with that. Life has a lot to offer besides growing inordinately large muscles. And once one has accepted the fact that there are some genetic facts that cannot be changed, something else happens—the training angst that many suffer will disappear and one no longer will become frustrated or surprised at the modest muscular results that one's bodybuilding efforts might bring forth. The best analogy I can find to put this situation into context is the following:

Instead of humans, think of another animal species; let's say horses. Within this species there exists considerable genetic differentiation, and yet, despite this great differentiation, there is also the commonality of the species (they are "horses" after all). One sect of this differentiation is the Quarter Horse, which is an average-size horse. Another is the Clydesdale, which is a truly massive horse renowned for its power and physique. Now let us imagine a scenario whereby a large portion of young male Quarter Horses desire to become bigger horses. They aren't fully grown yet, but in looking at the adult Quarter Horses they see only average-sized animals, only slightly bigger than themselves. Then one day they see a Clydesdale—and their world changes. That's what they want to look like! To their delight they discover that there is a magazine that specializes on the activities of Clydesdale horses called *Big Horse Monthly*. Inside the pages of this publication are featured pictures exclusively of Clydesdales and, seeing as there is a dollar to be made, certain of the Clydesdales, along with the publisher of the magazine, recognize that a large enough segment of the Quarter Horse community really wants to become big like Clydesdales are. So within the pages of the magazine they sell special foodstuffs (oats) that the Clydesdale eats and also sell exercise programs that the Clydesdales claim resulted in making them bigger and stronger. The young Quarter Horses might well think to themselves, *Wow! Those Clydesdales weren't always that big—and yet look at them now! I'm going to purchase one of those courses, and their special brand of oats, so that I can become big and strong like them.* So he purchases a particular Clydesdale's training course, and when that doesn't give him the results he wants, he buys another course from another Clydesdale featured in the magazine. He reads that one particular Clydesdale eats a lot of oats and pulls beer wagons around several days a week. *Eureka!* thinks the Quarter Horse, *That's what I'm going to do! I'm going to start eating a lot of oats and pull beer wagons around so I can look like him!* So he eats more oats than he needs and does his best to pull around beer wagons. After a month of this he is fatter (from eating more than his physiology requires) and his joints ache and his muscles are inflamed from doing too much work for his physiology—and, worst of all (to him), he still looks like a Quarter Horse and not a Clydesdale. Of course, the reason why he couldn't pull off the transformation isn't a lack of willingness to train hard or to eat what he thinks is required, but rather the simple fact that he doesn't possess the genetic disposition that makes a Clydesdale a Clydesdale.

And so it is with young human males who subscribe to muscle magazines and look at pictures of bodybuilders that have a greater genetic predisposition for growing larger muscles than they do. They are free to copy what the bodybuilders do in terms of training and duplicating what they eat, but those bodybuilders will always be the Clydesdales of our species and the young men will always be the Quarter Horses. And this will remain the case no matter how much time and money they invest in training, training equipment, or nutritional programs.

THE PROTEIN ISSUE

As touched upon in the previous pages, genetics is an area that the body-building industry doesn't really talk much about because there's no return on it. False implications go a long way in bodybuilding, as all training courses and supplement sales are predicated on the belief that the results of the genetically exceptional can be yours by purchasing such products. Within the pages (both online and print) of these same muscle magazines, those seeking to build bigger muscles will not only find articles allegedly written by certain champion bodybuilders detailing how they trained in order to develop their muscles but also, in page after page, the young readers will be inundated with a barrage of subtle (and not-so-subtle) advertisements for various powders and pills to maximize whatever growth their gym sessions might be stimulating. Of course, the

magazines seldom tell their young readers that champion bodybuilders also take growth hormones and anabolic steroid drugs to make their
muscles grow to such large proportions. They also seldom mention the
damage such long-term ingestion of these anabolic agents can have on the
hearts, livers, and endocrine systems of those who abuse such drugs over
a long period of time. And why would they lower themselves to report
on the health hazards of such drugs? Particularly when they aren't in the
health business, they're in the supplement business. As far as they're concerned, your health is your concern—not theirs. *Caveat emptor.*

While all nutritional scientists would agree on the need for adequate protein in one's diet for all-around health, few would agree with
the inordinate emphasis this macronutrient has received from faddists
and protein hucksters over the decades for its role in building muscle.
Protein has been a best-selling supplement for decades, with most people
advised to take it after a workout to allow their muscles to build up bigger and stronger. However, when this prescription was scrutinized more
carefully it was discovered that taking a protein supplement immediately
after working out did *nothing.*[7] Then there is the issue of quality control in
the protein supplement industry. Indeed, a recent investigation of several
leading protein supplements revealed that many of these protein powders
actually lacked protein![8]

Certainly a lack of protein in what is supposed to be a protein supplement should be a red flag for consumers, but what's even more alarming
is when one is consuming a bodybuilding supplement that one believes
will make him stronger and healthier only to learn that scientists have
now discovered a link between it and testicular cancer.[9] This was the finding of a study that concluded that men who took popular bodybuilding
supplements such as creatine or androstenedione were shown to have up
to a 177 percent higher chance of developing testicular cancer than men
who didn't—and the risk was worse if they started the supplementation
while they were young. Earlier research on androstenedione indicated
that it could damage the testes. According to epidemiologist and study-
leader Tongzhang Zheng of Brown University, "The observed relationship was strong . . . If you used at an earlier age, you had a higher risk. If
you used them longer, you had a higher risk. If you used multiple types,
you had a higher risk."[10] The study indicated that the men who took a

muscle-building supplement had on average a 65 percent greater risk of developing testicular cancer than those who didn't. This risk increased to 177 percent if the men used more than one type of bodybuilding supplement.

What has given the bodybuilding supplement manufacturers (most notably the ones who manufactured various protein products) traction over the decades is that all efforts to build "bigger muscles" have focused primarily on muscle *tissue*, per se, rather than on other components within that same tissue that have a greater bearing upon increasing the size of a given muscle. By far the largest component responsible for a muscle's size is how much water it stores.

When most young men begin their bodybuilding training, they notice that their bodies' response to such training is (in as much as there will be a response at all) much quicker during the first several months than it is afterward. There is an initial palpable change in the size of their muscles that gives them confidence that they are on the right track and that many hope will continue until their muscles reach the size they are hoping to attain. However, the perceived size increases one experiences early in one's training career are not a result of a building up of muscle tissue (i.e., the "protein" component of muscle), per se, but rather has been attributed to edema or swelling (water retention) within one's muscles, resulting from minor damage occurring[11] largely as a consequence of their muscles being introduced to the novelty of resistance training.

This really shouldn't be surprising as, despite the persistent din from supplement manufacturers that muscles are made of protein and, therefore, one seeking to build up the size of their muscles can't consume enough of this macronutrient, the facts of the matter are that only 22 percent of a muscle is comprised of protein. The remaining composition is 70 percent water and 6 to 8 percent lipids and inorganic material. Protein is only a small component of muscle tissue, but its importance has been overemphasized in muscle magazines over the years because the protein manufacturers recognized long ago that they couldn't sell you water that you can get for free out of your kitchen faucet.

Once one understands this, if bigger muscles is your goal it becomes obvious that you will be better served by looking into the mechanism that causes your muscles to retain or store water. The use of certain "muscle-building" drugs, such as synthol, an injectable oil, has grotesquely demonstrated just how important water is to this process as, once injected, synthol produces a fantastic amount of water retention in a muscle, owing to the phenomenon of inflammation that occurs in its presence. Little to no building of actual muscle "tissue" takes place in such instances, but the muscle that the synthol is injected into morphs into elephantine proportions.

Unlike myostatin, which places a regulator on how much actual muscle tissue one can build, no such governor exists with regard to water retention, which is why the bodybuilders who inject their muscles with irritants such as synthol create extreme inflammation/water retention, and produce ridiculous if not grotesque increases in the size of their muscles. Even certain classes of anabolic steroids have been known for their water-retaining effect. So the more water you can store in your muscles, the bigger they will be.

Consequently, when one shifts one's focus from protein to the mechanism that allows water to be stored in muscle, we note that one of the biggest factors influencing this phenomenon is glycogen. Water bonds with glycogen at a rate of three grams of water to every one gram of glycogen, and the muscle fibers that store the most glycogen happen to be the Fast-Twitch fibers—the highest energy output fibers in the body. So, if you want to build bigger muscles, then you will want to tap the glycogen out of the fibers that store the most of it, which again requires very high-energy output, and, which in turn, will cause the muscle fibers that have emptied their glycogen stores to overcompensate by storing even more glycogen[12] (and, thus, more water) in those same muscles, thereby increasing the volume or size of the muscles you are training.

PART THREE
EXERCISE—A NEW PARADIGM

CHAPTER TEN

THE GENETIC FACTOR

Picture yourself in line for a ride at an amusement park. It's a long line and it's a hot day. An hour passes before you reach the gate that separates you from the ride. Once you reach the gate a superintendent comes out to tell you that you're not allowed on the ride, as you don't meet the minimum height requirements. You might well be angered by this, coming as it did at the last possible minute, but being angry isn't going to change the fact. It is what it is and you simply will not be able to experience the ride.

Disappointed, you move on, but you are still a little agitated. If only somebody had come up to you before you had gotten into line and waited all that time and said, "This ride isn't for you. There is a minimum height requirement for it, and you don't meet it. They won't let you on." You might been very grateful if you had received this news up front, as it would have saved you all of the time and frustration that you experienced standing in line only to be turned away. Well, in the field of exercise, I'd like to be that "somebody" for you. This ride called exercise has its own set of genetic restrictions, and you may not meet the entry requirements.

Individuals seeking to improve themselves over the past three decades have purchased millions of copies of exercise and diet books and DVDs. Many of these individuals believe themselves to be lacking something, and if they could just pinpoint that missing element (be it nutritional or exercise-related) they will then have the means to transform themselves into something other than what they are presently. Such beliefs and the media that feeds them are the oil that greases the wheels of the fitness industry.

The idea that one can look or perform like a superstar athlete or celebrity simply by aping his or her workout or nutritional program or by using such a person's brand of baseball or hockey equipment is what generates tens of millions of dollars of supplemental income for athletes during their careers, and what makes the Board of Directors at huge corporations such as Rawlings, C.C.M., and Bauer very happy. Additionally, while good equipment is nice to have and certain training programs can represent a refreshing change of pace, the fact is that you and I, and our existing skill sets, simply can't morph into those of someone else, particularly when that someone else possesses a genetic gift that we do not have.

The exceptional (i.e., those in possession of a rare skill for a given athletic event such as soccer) are, by definition, not indicative of the norm in such matters, which is precisely why these people are exceptional. You can drink all the Gatorade you want, but doing so will never endow you with the skill set for hockey that Sidney Crosby has. In addition, and particularly when it comes to the realm of training, many world-class athletes are not above misleading either the general public or their followers. You may recall that the once-revered road cyclist Lance Armstrong proclaimed that, "Everybody wants to know what I'm on. What am I *on*? I'm on my bike busting my ass six hours a day." It turned out that Lance was also on steroids, testosterone, growth hormone, E.P.O., and cortisone (which is what allowed him to bust his ass on a bike for six hours a day). Such deception and subterfuge is really not that surprising when big-money endorsements are at stake; after all, these are athletes we're talking about, not saints.

I always try to impress upon my personal training clients the fact that they must form a realistic assessment of their own genetic gifts and limitations if they don't want their exercise endeavor to leave them chronically frustrated. If purchasing the same brand of golf clubs used by a PGA star such as Tiger Woods could imbue you with his skill set for the game of golf, then there would no longer be anything exceptional about Tiger; it would be the clubs he used that made him so great. In addition, every local golf course would be full of comparative talent as a result of its members using the same clubs that Tiger does. Though I'm not one to rain on anybody's enthusiasm (unless it is grossly misplaced), the reality is that most of us don't possess such exceptional physical attributes. We're "normal," part of the great mediocrity; firmly entrenched in the ranks of the physically average. We may even be below average—but that's okay. Being average means that we have all the qualities that are necessary to survive and even be successful. We just aren't in possession of that one exceptional physical attribute that is of such rarity that a lot of people would be willing to pay money to see it on display or that big corporations would be willing to provide us with huge sums of money in order to align it with their products. And while I would be the first to tell you that you need to be fit so that you can more fully experience all that life has to offer, and that you need to be healthy enough to be able to function optimally, the cold hard truth is that you can obtain these rather modest goals without ever driving a golf ball 400 yards, running a 10K, winning a Stanley Cup, lifting double your bodyweight, or winning the heavyweight division of the UFC.

It should be emphasized that the training that exceptional athletes can engage in is simply a demonstration of what the genetically exceptional can do. Not sharing these same physical attributes, being non-exceptional in other words, we should not be frustrated with the fact that we cannot demonstrate like abilities either on the playing field or in the gymnasium. Lions don't exhibit the same leaping ability as gazelles, nor do they exhibit the tree-climbing ability of monkeys, but they don't seem to be losing too much sleep over it. Still, as Voltaire once wrote, "It is difficult to free fools from the chains they revere." And while the famous philosopher wrote this about religion, I've learned over the years that discussing exercise with some people is not dissimilar to discussing religion or politics; that is, many people hold fast to their views about exercise and the benefits they believe they derive from performing it, very often embracing them all the more passionately in an inverse ratio to the validity of such viewpoints.

I will admit to having a certain kind of empathy for those who hold fast to their fitness industry model of exercise, as I did too at one point. Back in the mid-1970s, Arnold Schwarzenegger was the biggest thing to ever hit bodybuilding. He had won all of the top bodybuilding titles convincingly (with the exception of his Mr. Olympia victory in 1980—but that is another story entirely), and was featured on the covers of all of the muscle magazines of the day. He appeared in ads endorsing many of the nutritional and exercise equipment products of his employer Joe Weider, and personally sold tens of thousands of training courses in which he advocated that one should train upwards of six days a week, twice a day, for two hours a workout and 20 sets per body part. Thousands of us attempted to train in Arnold's fashion, but nothing in the way of Arnold-like muscles ever sprouted on our bodies. Now, over 30 years later, we still don't see a lot of Arnolds running around, despite the fact that his training methods have been published in even more books, revealed on DVDs, and are still being featured in the current muscle magazines. No, Arnold's muscular success came through two other avenues: steroid use (which he has gone on record as using) and a genetic predisposition for building inordinately large muscles.

To use another example, give me a call when you set Lance Armstrong's record for Tour de France victories. You'll forgive me if I don't hold my breath waiting for that call. Armstrong, like all other great athletes, had the genetic predisposition to be the most successful road-racing cyclist in history. And while other road-racing cyclists have utilized his training method, none have come close to equaling his competitive successes.

The best example of a complete non-transference of an elite athlete's skills might well involve hockey legend Wayne Gretzky. I recall being in France when I was 12 years old for a family skiing vacation. I was a huge hockey fan at the time and wandered into a bookstore in the town of Courchevel, where to my surprise I spied a French language hockey magazine. On the cover were the words: "Wayne Gretzky Peewee Sensation!" In other words, he was a hockey phenomenon even at peewee age and people from as far away as France knew about him and his prodigious talent. (To sidetrack for a moment, could you imagine having been Gretzky's Peewee coach once Wayne hit the big time and began shattering NHL scoring records? That coach could have hung up a shingle indicating his role in Gretzky's minor hockey development—particularly if he came out with this information at the height of Gretzky's career—and he would have made a fortune by training other peewee-aged kids in Canada and the United States. Presumably, Gretzky's Peewee coach trained Gretzky no differently than he did any of the other players on Gretzky's Peewee team, but only Gretzky would go on to become the greatest player in hockey history). Given Gretzky's phenomenal career, it may be natural to assume that he must have picked up some tricks and secrets that were directly responsible for his becoming so phenomenally successful. And, indeed, he might well have. However, some time after Gretzky retired from playing professional hockey he became a head coach in the National Hockey League (NHL). This presented him with a formidable opportunity to share his tricks and secrets that resulted in his being such a prodigious talent to an entire team, which should have resulted in his icing a championship team of Gretzky-like talent. However, when Gretzky was the coach of the Phoenix Coyotes in the NHL and the players under his charge had the benefit of learning all of his training methods, tips, and secrets firsthand from the man himself, the result was that they finished dead last in their division and failed to produce even one player that came close to the talent of Wayne Gretzky. The reason, alas, is that athletic success is a kingdom where genetics always wears the crown.

The huge genetic component of athletic success cannot be overstated. Indeed, a study that was conducted by Grand Valley State University that examined the role of genetics on sprinters, tells the tale:

> Most scientists agree that expertise requires both innate talent and proper training. Nevertheless, the highly influential deliberate practice model (DPM) of expertise holds that either talent does not exist, or that its contribution to performance differences is negligible. It predicts that initial performance will be unrelated to achieving expertise and that a long period of deliberate practice—at least 10 years or 10,000 hours—is necessary and sufficient for achieving expertise. We tested these predictions in the domain of sprinting. Study 1 reviewed the biographies of 15 Olympic sprint champions. Study 2 reviewed the biographies of the 20 fastest male sprinters in U.S. history. In all documented cases, *sprinters were exceptional prior to or coincident with their initiation of formal training* [italics mine]. Furthermore, most reached world-class status rapidly (Study 1 median = 3 years; Study 2 median = 7.5). Study 3 surveyed U.S. national collegiate championships qualifiers in sprints and throws. Sprinters

recalled being faster as youths than did throwers, whereas throwers recalled greater strength and overhand throwing ability. Sprinters' best performances in their first season of high school, generally the onset of formal training, were consistently faster than 95-99% of their peers. Collectively, these results falsify the DPM for sprinting. Because speed is foundational for many sports, they challenge the DPM generally.[1]

The great athletes that populate our sporting world are wonderful examples of the power of random genetic variation self-selecting for those activities in which they happen to excel. In other words, exceptional athletes have a genetic advantage that allows them to perform certain neuromuscular activities that are required in order to excel at a given sport better than most other people. This is what makes them so exceptional in a given athletic event—as opposed to their training programs being the sole reason for their level of athletic success. Indeed, the individual who runs the hockey school I cited in an earlier chapter had his best seasons in the NHL *prior to* his engaging in a more zealous off-ice "conditioning" program (the same one that he's now charging young players $13,000 a week for). And the reason should now be coming more clearly into focus. Great athletes are largely the result of random genetic chance; the training and dietary regimens they choose to employ have much less to do with their ultimate success than did their "choosing" the right parents. This is not to dismiss the role of proper diet and exercise in an athlete's success, but rather to quantify it more accurately as coming in at a distant second to genetics. Consequently, if your desires are not firmly rooted in genetic reality, you may very well end up frustrated and disappointed.

This being said, many people fear genetics, or rather fear what their genetics might bring into being. While such a fear is justified when applied to many of the diseases (such as cancer) that can lie dormant within an individual for many years before suddenly appearing as a life-threatening manifestation, it is quite often unjustified when applied to cosmetic issues such as how large one's muscles might become. Strength training, for example, is without question one of the most productive activities that one can engage in from a health and fitness standpoint, and yet it remains true that there are many women who presently avoid it for fear that they will end up looking like the current Mr. Olympia. On the other side of the coin, there are many men who once engaged in strength training but ended up quitting in frustration because they didn't end up looking like the current Mr. Olympia. In the case of women, such fears are unfounded (recall the role of myostatin, among other genetic requirements to develop large muscles), and for men, such frustration as they experience is typically the norm for the same reasons, along with the simple fact that being able to build exceptionally large muscles is a very rare trait in human beings generally. And it just so happens that those who have a larger than normal musculature are better suited to sports and activities that having larger muscles gives them a distinct advantage in, such as weight lifting, bodybuilding, and certain track and field events. But these people don't have big muscles simply because they lifted weights; they gravitated to activities such as lifting weights because they already had bigger than normal muscles, which gave them a distinct advantage in such activities. Bouncing a basketball will not make one seven feet tall, but one who is seven feet tall will gravitate toward sports such as basketball where such inordinate height offers a distinct advantage.

In the case of one having bigger muscles, such individuals gravitate toward activities such as bodybuilding where those who are particularly muscular will be popularized and utilized for marketing purposes in bodybuilding and fitness publications, where they are often lionized with the underlying implication that their appearance is "possible for anyone." However, the marketing implication is what makes for the fear in many women that they, too, will end up looking like that, and results in the chronic frustration experienced by many men who, despite lifting weights many days per week, never will.

Nevertheless, the late-night infomercials continue to flicker across our television screens and their announcers proclaim in an adrenalized but matter-of-fact voice: "Now YOU can build sleek biceps, a sexy core, and sculpted legs." This is said over B-roll footage of someone with completely different genetics than most of us displaying his or her single-digit bodyfat levels along with these well-developed body parts. Then a person comes on camera and delivers a testimonial about how he or she lost weight, built muscle, and how the opposite sex is now giving him or her sly winks. If you're honest, there's a part of you that really wants to buy into this concept—i.e., that you can transform yourself and essentially look like somebody exceptional. You're not alone. Sales of infomercial fitness products (which pretty much all use the same format) are through the roof. Nautilus™, the company that once created a hugely popular line of commercial exercise equipment (back in the 1970s and '80s), not too long ago purchased Bowflex™, a home exercise infomercial product. The sales of Bowflex™ went through the roof as a result of their infomercials on television, which surprised everyone at the Nautilus company so much that for a time Nautilus dropped its commercial line of exercise equipment altogether in order to focus its attention on where its real money was being made—the Bowflex™ infomercial product.

As awesome as these infomercials were, the reality is that the old adage remains true that you cannot turn a sow's ear into a silk purse, no matter what exercise equipment or protocol you use. I have a 60-year-old client who was about to quit coming to my facility after a year of training because she didn't have a "butt like Jennifer Lopez." Another middle-aged woman was quite upset because she wanted to have "abs like Janet Jackson." So prevalent is the assumption that if you just employ the right exercises (or the right equipment) in your workouts, you will then somehow be able to alter your DNA, and profoundly impact your body's appearance. Again, not to rain on anybody's parade, but I've never seen anybody exercise his or her way out of his or her genetics. Yes, you can lose body fat and, yes, again, you can build muscle, but it is very hard to lose a lot of the former and almost impossible to build a lot of the latter. However, if you can do both to some degree, then you will most certainly have created a dramatic difference for the better in your appearance, but a Mr. Olympia physique or a "JLo butt" are predominantly the result of muscle fiber density, and that is a genetically inherited trait. You can stimulate the fibers in your muscles to grow larger, but if you only have 400,000 fibers in a given muscle as compared to someone else who has 800,000, then you will only have half the number of fibers available to make bigger and your size in that region will always—even at best—be half that of those who have more fibers in their respective muscles to stimulate into growth.

Ditto for the "Janet Jackson abs" (which she herself doesn't seem to be able to hold onto very well). Janet may well have a naturally fast metabolism, or have starved herself to achieve such a high level of definition, or had a personal trainer who gave her some chemical assistance to help amp her metabolism and build muscle. And don't make the mistake of thinking that celebrities, who often play morally upright individuals in their movies and TV series, are above taking some contraband to achieve a certain look. There once was, and perhaps still is, a personal trainer in California that I knew who told me that he put one of his celebrity clients on steroids to help her achieve a certain muscular look that she displayed in a certain film. This guy was more accurately a drug peddler than a personal trainer, but of course the look that his client obtained was then claimed to be solely the result of his expertise in guiding her nutrition practices and workouts in the gym. As a result, he soon had a list of celebrities that went to him for his personal training services because he was capable of creating "that look" in his clients. The public was led to believe that the actress he trained achieved this look through diligent hard work in the gym and being on a strict diet. And while these elements did have something to do with the look the actress displayed, very potent anabolic drugs were responsible for the lion's share of her cosmetic transformation.

If your health is important to you and you're not willing to risk your long-term health by taking muscle-building drugs, then you're left with the best that you can do with the cards that nature dealt to you at birth— and this can only be realized by exercising hard and dieting.

Furthermore, if having "Janet Jackson abs" is your goal, then train hard to develop your abdominal muscles. And if having them stand out on your abdomen in bold relief is important to you, diet for a sufficiently long period of time (perhaps six months) to bring about this condition. Then enjoy it for about a week, for that's about as long as you will be able to endure the dieting and deprivation necessary to achieve that look. And even then your abs may never look anything like Janet Jackson's (or anybody else's), as not everyone's abdominal muscles possess the same shape. Indeed, not everyone has the genetics to create a "six pack"; some will develop four packs, some eight packs, others (those with less muscle fiber density in their abdominal muscles) won't develop any "packs" at all, but will simply have a flatter abdomen with no discernable ridges. It comes down to the length of the muscle belly and the fibers per cubic inch that the muscle group in question possesses, which, again, is a matter of genetic endowment and not subject to alteration through exercise.

And if you think that doing a lot of direct abdominal work, such as daily sessions of sit-ups, will burn more fat in the belly region, you might want to think again. A study that was conducted to see what effect direct abdominal exercise had on melting body fat from the abdominal area revealed that, after six weeks of five days per week direct abdominal workouts, those that trained their abs in such a dedicated fashion lost no more fat from their midsection than did the control group who performed "zero" direct abdominal work.[2]

For the same reason that we don't all share the same height, or possess the same eye color, the same hair texture, and the same skin pigment, we don't all share the same genetics for leanness, muscle size, and shape. Remember, being you is an okay thing to be. In fact it's the best thing you can be, so why not be the fittest and healthiest you that your genetics will allow?

CHAPTER ELEVEN

THE CONSERVATION OF ENERGY PHENOMENON (C.E.P.)

There was a period during our species' history when our ancestors would sporadically engage in a type of effort that would engage their high-energy (Fast-Twitch) muscle fibers simply as a result of living in a hostile environment.

Over the centuries, however, we slowly succeeded in making our environment far less hostile, but our doing so resulted in the creation of a new environment in which the fibers that can play a huge role in the preservation of our health (Fast-Twitch fibers) are being allowed to languish and atrophy. They have languished not because we're lazy (as is often asserted) but because we are strongly and biologically disinclined to output large amounts of energy unless doing so is absolutely necessary for our continued survival. And it's important, at least within the context of exercise, to understand just why this is.

SURVIVAL & THE CONSERVATION OF ENERGY

We are a species that has hardwired into its cells a strong impulse to conserve energy, owing to the fact that this act of conserving energy is what has allowed our species to survive over the millenniums. The prospect of starvation was a very real (and often a daily) threat to our species right up until the turn of the last century. Indeed, in some sections of our globe the threat of securing adequate food to sustain human existence still persists to this day. Surviving in such an environment for tens of thousands of years resulted in two energy-related attitudes forming in us; the first being that if you didn't have to output energy, don't do it because you may not be able to get it back from the environment; and the second being that if you happen upon an energy source, consume it—because it may not be there tomorrow. As energy (nutrition) is what keeps our cells alive, and as we are little more than a collection of these cells, you can well understand why energy acquisition and preservation are the top priorities on the biological list of things we must do to survive. You can quit smoking and you can quit drinking alcohol, but you'll never quit eating—and live.

Fast-forwarding from our food-deprived ancestors to present day, these same two attitudes of energy acquisition and preservation still predominate within not only our psyches, but also our somas—the only difference now being that we find ourselves living in an environment where sources of energy are omnipresent. We have lots of food in our homes, more food is available in grocery stores and fastfood restaurants (that are often accessible within minutes from where we work and live), and then there are the omnipresent vending machines inside our workplaces and schools. Our biology is such that we still have these very strong impulses to consume these sources of energy when given the opportunity, and there are few among us who can (and do) resist such strong biological urges.

On the flip side of the coin, we also have lots of choices to compete for our energy output options when it comes to exercise and, given the above, it's little wonder that we naturally tend to gravitate toward low-energy output activities rather than high-energy output activities. Psychologically, we sense that we must maintain something of a balance between our energy input and energy output, but not knowing how much energy we typically input into our systems, nor the energy output differential between our various classes of muscle fibers, most of us simply prefer not to expend much in the way of mental calories thinking about it. We simply assume that "using our muscles" to perform an activity is using all of its fibers and that almost any type of physical activity that involves our muscles is "exercise," and therefore "good" for us. And when we weigh our options in this regard, we quickly discern that some types of muscular work are unpleasant (hard, difficult, high-energy output, etc.) and leave us feeling exhausted, winded, and perhaps even sore, while other types of muscular work are far more pleasant and don't leave us feeling any of these things. And so it should come as no surprise that we are far more inclined to prefer low-energy output activities such as a brisk walk or some mild stretching, than we are a fast run or lifting weights.

Given our present environment of energy abundance, most of us are destined to become fat and unhealthy by giving in to these impulses to input as much energy as available and output as little energy as possible.

We rationalize this predilection for low-energy output activity by the words we choose to describe it: stimulating, relaxing, easy, effortless, and, my personal favorite, "more natural." The more demanding energy output activity we classify as hard, demanding, unpleasant, painful, straining, and "unnatural." However, when viewed in the proper context, we are actually saying:

"Hard" = High Effort

High Effort = High-Energy Output

High-Energy Output = Tapping Glycolytic fibers (Fast-Twitch Fibers)

Tapping Glycolytic fibers = Glycogen being emptied out of your muscles at a great rate

As you can see, tapping high-energy fibers is not a bad thing. I've already indicated the health benefits that can be obtained by tapping our Fast-Twitch Fibers, the class of muscle fibers that happen to store the most glycogen, but doing so will also ensure that you have tapped all of the lower order of fibers as well, which includes all of the metabolic pathways that serve each class of these fibers. Lower intensity activities (such as walking) simply do not tap more than one class of muscle fiber and it happens to be the one that contains the least amount of glycogen and, thus, activities that require only these fibers have a minimal effect on our long-term health.

What you perceive as being "hard work" is more aptly titled "high-energy output activity." And contrary to our natural preference for low-energy output activity, high-energy output activity is actually the safest. The reasons for this are twofold; first, more demanding muscular work simply cannot be carried on for as long as less demanding muscular work, which thereby reduces the volume of wear and tear that can be brought to bear on our joints and connective tissues; second, your body will normally only tap high-energy fibers in a flight-or-fight situation (think of them as the nitrous oxide that we pour on our engines to get us safely away from trouble should trouble arise) and, consequently, our bodies have set up a lot of internal safety measures to allow the muscles (and the energy that fuels them) to do their job of delivering you from harm in a safe and efficient manner. In this case, certain stress hormones are released that cause the aperture of the arteries to expand (or vasodilate), thus saving your heart from having to pump harder in order to circulate your blood to your working muscles. In addition, muscles contracting intensely serve as auxiliary pumps to assist in this increased circulation of the blood, which is something that lower energy output activity simply doesn't do. With lower energy output activity the demand for more oxygenated blood is present, but not the means by which to deliver it with less stress to your heart and vascular system. The heart's only option in these situations is to pump harder and more frequently, which, if you happen to have a weak arterial wall can prove fatal, as the mortality rate of occasional snow-shovelers and weekend athletes will attest.

The reality is that one needn't be afraid of exercising "too hard," as long as your time spent engaging in such exercise is brief. Apart from being a very safe form of exercise for your heart, high-energy output work also taps your body's most important fibers (Fast-Twitch), which are absolutely vital for realizing our primary health and fitness goals such as lowering blood pressure, reducing cholesterol levels, and diminishing our chance of contracting diabetes. Rather than fearing muscular exhaustion—i.e., the temporary emptying of the energy (ATP and glycogen) supplies within muscles—this "emptying of the gas tank" is the sine qua non of any meaningful exercise program, but it requires engineering such an exercise program to ensure that the activation of Fast-Twitch (i.e., high-energy) muscle fibers takes place.

Fast-Twitch fibers also happen to be the ones that begin to atrophy first as we age. The burning sensation (caused by lactic acidosis) that attends the use of Fast-Twitch fibers is what typically dissuades people from exercise protocols that engage them. However, the burning sensation that one experiences when tapping these fibers is not something bad to be avoided, but simply a part of your biology that you should learn to make your peace with. Think of lactic acid as the exhaust that is emitted from more powerful engines. When you engage Slow-Twitch fibers you are engaging very small engines that don't produce much in the way of exhaust. When you tap Intermediate-Twitch fibers you will be engaging slightly bigger engines that will produce a level of exhaust that is perceptible (i.e., a mild burning sensation). And when you tap Fast-Twitch fibers you will be engaging your most powerful metabolic engines and they simply emit a greater amount of exhaust (perceived as a burning sensation) than the preceding two classes of fibers. In addition, from a cardiovascular perspective, lactic acid can be said to be the "coal" of the aerobic furnace, as lactic acid is the chemical compound that your body converts to an enzyme called pyruvate, and pyruvate is what engages the mitochondria within your cells and causes your aerobic machinery to cycle at its highest capacity.

While the majority of clients that I have trained over the years understand why they train in a high-energy output manner, there are some who have never grasped the "whys" and "wherefores" of the process. These are typically the clients that will not stay with any exercise program very long and eventually drop out, citing that "it's too hard." However, exercise, as we've seen, must be perceived as "hard," as what we interpret as being "hard" the body simply accepts as high-energy output activity. And high-energy output activity is where all the gold that can be panned from exercise is to be found.

It must be pointed out that exercise, per se, is nothing more than a stimulus that acts upon our bodies. That stimulus must cause a sufficient drain of the muscles' energy reserves to cause the body to protect itself and its reserves against potential future assaults of like severity, and it does this by making an adaptive response by either increasing the size of its muscle tissue or the energy supplies that fuel the muscle (and occasionally it increases both of these factors). These responses take place while the body is at rest (the time in between exercise sessions) as, obviously, it cannot replenish energy that is being used up concomitantly. And this is why the recovery interval (i.e., the time off in between workouts) is so crucially important.

THE CONSERVATION OF ENERGY PHENOMENON (C.E.P.)

Often what people take to be an improvement in their fitness level is, in reality, simply the body learning how to perform a given activity with less muscular/energy output and, thus, less involvement/improvement of one's muscular and cardiovascular system. It needs to be pointed out that everything you do, from learning how to walk to running your first 10K, is a skill set that the body needs time and practice to adjust to. Initially, not being familiar with the requirements of the activity, the body will tackle it head on with everything it's got. The body doesn't know that you are doing the activity for recreational purposes or to improve your fitness level; all it knows is that its energy output requirements have suddenly spiked and that its survival might hinge on its ability to immediately meet these requirements in order to get you out of the situation that has suddenly caused a demand for more energy.

After repeated exposure to the same activity, however, the body begins to more critically assess the activity being performed in terms of its energy requirements and in terms of the precise amount of muscular involvement that is minimally necessary to accomplish the task. Eventually the body learns to perform the activity in a manner that requires far less muscle fiber involvement (and thus far less energy output) by keying in on precisely how many fibers are required at precisely what time in the movement and then proceeds to act on this calculus by reducing the involvement of muscle fibers and energy supplies that it views to be superfluous to the performance of the activity. This happens after repeated exposure to the said activity, resulting in the heart and lungs having to service the working of much less muscle tissue and our bodies not burning as much energy (calories) as they did when we performed the activity initially. Soon the same activity fails to stimulate the same biological response (which in this case would be the maximum recruitment of muscle fibers), and if one then wishes to have one's body repeat that original metabolic response, the activity must somehow be altered. In the case of running, the run must be made longer, performed at a quicker pace, or an alternate terrain must be selected that is in some way different from what one has grown accustomed to. When this happens, the original "all-in" response returns.

However, if one is not aware of this phenomenon, one might mistakenly confuse this economization of energy and muscle fiber recruitment by the body as a sign of cardiovascular improvement. After all, when one starts running (even after a moderate hiatus) the effect is profound: the heart beats like a trip hammer, perspiration flows freely, muscles and joints ache the next day, and one is breathing heavily during the performance of the activity (and for many minutes afterward). A month later, however, that same run produces very few of the effects that had been felt so acutely the month before. Now the heartbeat barely rises above a base line, the sweat is modest, and the next day there exist little to no signs that one ran at all the day before. Some change has obviously happened, and at first blush it would appear that one's fitness and aerobic capacity has improved rather dramatically. However, as we've just seen, what has really happened is that the body is now investing less of its energy into the activity. Initially the runner's body may have sent 90 percent of its musculature into action, but over time it realized that if a slight alteration in the timing of the recruitment of muscle fibers was made, it could still perform the required activity with a lot less muscle fibers being involved and, thus, a lot less energy expended. Consequently, the signs that running is becoming easier (i.e., not breathing as hard at the end of the run, traveling a greater distance before being overcome by fatigue, etc.) don't necessarily indicate that there is a strengthening of the runner's cardiovascular system taking place. What it might actually be representing is a gradual diminishment of the demands that are being placed upon his or her cardiovascular system from when he or she first returned to the activity one month earlier. I have christened this phenomenon the Conservation of Energy Phenomenon (C.E.P.).

If you think about it, this syndrome manifests during every physical activity in which we opt to engage. It was present the first time we ever drove a car with a standard (not automatic) transmission; i.e., every muscle was tense, we were sweating, and our pulse rate was elevated. But a month or so later we found ourselves zipping down the highway, singing along with a song on the radio with one hand on the steering wheel. Again, there was "zero" improvement in our muscular or cardiovascular system in this example; our bodies simply learned how to execute this activity with far less muscular involvement than before and, therefore, far less energy expenditure.

Moreover, if sweating, muscular fatigue, and an elevated pulse rate were the sine qua non symptoms of having had a cardiovascular workout, then your first time behind the wheel of a standard automobile might well meet that criteria. What has transpired in both scenarios, however, is the C.E.P.; i.e., a refinement in motor unit selection and sequencing that allows one to do the same activity (external performance) with less (internal performance). The important thing for you to take away from this is not so much *why* this happens (unless you get off on reading about biochemistry and evolutionary biology) but rather the understanding *that* it happens. And, as indicated, there is no physical activity that is exempt from its influence—even walking. An article in the *Los Angeles Times* by columnist Melissa Healy reported on a study on walkers that confirmed that our bodies always seek the path of less energy output:

> We may walk, run, swim or dance in a determined bid to burn off calories. But our bodies, obeying a more primitive impulse, are preserving energy at every turn. A study published . . . in the journal *Current Biology* finds that the evolutionary imperative of minimizing effort quite literally influences every step we take. The authors of the new study put people in robotic exoskeletons— wearable stepping aids that bristle with sensors and motors— and measured a key aspect of their gait (the frequency of their step) while the subjects walked on a treadmill. The researchers observed that pedestrians quickly and unconsciously find their preferred stride: the one that expends the least amount of energy per step. The researchers then used the intrusive robotic device to briefly perturb the subjects' step frequency. Initially, when walkers were unexpectedly nudged out of their comfort zone by the exoskeleton, they worked hard to maintain the stride they had established at the outset. That changed, though, when the researchers gave the subjects several minutes to explore different walking strategies on their own. When researchers started the treadmill again and resumed their measurements, the walkers immediately adopted major changes in their step frequency— shifting what had previously seemed like a natural preference. The result of the shift: They expended fewer calories than if they had persisted with their earlier gait. . . . Knocked repeatedly out of their comfort zones, subjects repeatedly adapted in ways that minimized their expenditure of calories. In terms of calories

unburned, the changes that subjects made to their gaits were very small: shifting to a new step frequency whittled calories expended, on average, by just 5%. But over a lifetime of walking, that adds up. And when you're exercising with the aim of burning maximum calories, it's a painful irony to be reminded that your body is working to thwart your efforts.[1]

The C.E.P. is one of the reasons I pay close attention to my clients' rate of respiration while I'm training them during a workout; if they are performing an exercise that previously had left them panting like a dog on a hot day but now seems to have no effect, then I know it's time to change the exercises they are doing, or the protocol they are using, as it is no longer recruiting the quantity of muscle fibers that it once did. Recall that Fast-Twitch fibers produce a mother load of lactic acid that is converted by the body to pyruvate, which is then processed through the aerobic system. The greater the rate of lactic acid production, I've found, the greater the aerobic effect. If you really want to experience an aerobic workout, make sure you are tapping Fast-Twitch fibers. And, as Fast-Twitch fibers are the fibers with the greatest potential to increase in size and strength, they are definitely the ones I want my clients engaging (along with the other lower order fibers for total metabolic health of course). So changing up the exercise protocol periodically is important in order to ensure that you are involving as many fibers as possible whenever one works out.

This was demonstrated clinically by researchers in Japan and the United States who noted that gains in muscle size are typically greater during the beginning stages of a person's training, then begin to taper out the more one is exposed to the same training stimulus. They sought to understand why this phenomenon occurred and discovered that the same training protocol performed over and over eventually resulted in the muscles becoming less sensitive to the training stimuli and that the motor (or neural) signaling necessary for an anabolic (or tissue-building) response to resistance exercise grew less sensitive to resistance exercise over time.[2] In some cases if the trainee took a protracted period of time off from training and then returned to his original protocol the original response returned to the same extent that it did previously. In other train-ees, however, taking time off from the same protocol that had been per-formed and then returning to it produced no effect at all.

The C.E.P. will also assert itself to thwart one's efforts to burn addi-tional calories if one adds more exercise to one's weekly routine. In a study reported in the journal *Current Biology*, it was determined that our body will further adjust to higher activity levels being imposed upon it in the very same manner in which it adapted to the reapplication of a more consistent stimulus; i.e., in both scenarios the body will reduce its energy output while performing the task at hand in an ongoing effort to conserve energy. This particular study examined 332 people from five different populations around the globe, consisting of those living in a township in South Africa, an agrarian population from Ghana, urban dwellers in Jamaica, suburban dwellers in the United States, and those who lived on an island in the Seychelles. Over the course of a week the researchers tracked the physical activity of their subjects through wear-able devices and measured their energy expenditure via a specialized urine test. The data revealed that while energy output did track upward with increased physical activity levels, it did so only up to a point. Beyond this point those who amped their physical activity levels above a modest baseline did not burn any additional calories.[3] One of the researchers, Amy Luke, a public health researcher at Loyola University in Chicago, probably wasn't too surprised by the finding, however, as she had pub-lished a paper in 2009 that compared overweight and obese women in the United States with lean women from rural Nigeria. At the time she had expected that the Nigerian women, being leaner, would have output more energy (i.e., burned more calories) on a daily basis as a result of their being more active. She was stunned, however, to learn that both groups of women burned the same number of calories and that the volume of exercise someone performed could not lead one to accurately predict weight change.[4] Her conclusion from this was that if you wanted to lose weight you would be better served to "eat fewer calories" than to try and output more energy via exercise.[5] Again, the C.E.P. is at play, and after countless millenniums, our bodies have become very good at figuring out ways to do all that we ask of them with the least amount of energy output possible. We must be aware of this phenomenon when we exercise, as even the most well-thought-out exercise program is not immune from our biological programming.

CHAPTER TWELVE

RESISTANCE TRAINING—
A BETTER WAY TO EXERCISE

Let us take a moment to recap what we have observed thus far. We note that exercise is always (in as much as movement is involved) a source of wear and tear (which is a bad thing). We also know that exercise can bring punishing amounts of force to the body (which is also a bad thing). And, to top it all off, exercise may have little to no effect upon the practitioner (a genetic thing). But we also know that if we don't do *something* to preserve our muscular function then we will lose it and, given that the life expectancy of our species is increasing, we don't want to spend the majority of our senior years with decreased functional ability, nor do we wish to suffer from the various health problems that attend a progressive loss of muscle mass.

Many of our species' health problems stem from the loss (over time) of our Fast-Twitch muscle fibers—the ones that store the most glycogen, and thus, the ones that have a direct bearing on issues such as type II diabetes, high blood pressure, high cholesterol levels, and cardiovascular disease. And while various forms of exercise can activate these fibers, the scientific research has concluded that only one type of exercise has emerged as being the safest and most beneficial way to engage them, and that exercise is resistance training.

THE CASE FOR RESISTANCE TRAINING

A 2006 article in the *Canadian Medical Association* (C.M.A.) *Journal* reported on a review of all of the evidence regarding the benefits of all forms of exercise. The researchers concluded that resistance training represented a:

paradigm shift . . . people with high levels of muscular strength have fewer functional limitations and lower incidences of chronic diseases such as diabetes, stroke, arthritis, coronary artery disease and pulmonary disorders . . . Musculoskeletal fitness is positively associated with functional independence, mobility, glucose homeostasis, bone health, psychological well being and overall quality of life and is negatively associated with the risk of falls, illness and premature death.[1]

Apart from the benefits the C.M.A. indicated above, resistance training is also the exercise of choice for the individual who has let go of such notions as "super health" and "miraculous transformations" and simply wants to achieve a realistic standard of fitness and muscular strength for him or herself that is both safe and sustainable. Resistance training engages one's muscles in a manner that involves as many metabolic pathways as possible, it requires the outputting of large amounts of energy when performed properly, and, at times, trips the growth and repair mechanism of the body into motion (I say "at times," as there is a genetic limit to one's ability to grow muscle), resulting in the individual trainee becoming stronger, healthier, and able to engage in enjoyable life activities that may not have been an option when the individual was weaker and less capable.

While other forms of exercise can also accomplish this objective (exercises such as running, cycling, swimming, gymnastics, rowing, and cross-country skiing come to mind), some of them (particularly in the case of running and cycling) only involve the muscles and metabolic pathways of the lower extremities. In addition, all of the activities mentioned bring a lot of wear and tear to one's body and require a considerable time investment. When the additional factor of safety is taken into consideration, resistance training emerges as, quite simply, the most rational choice when choosing an exercise modality. In a blog posted on his website (www.drmcguff.com) Doug McGuff, MD, indicated that proper resistance training delivered the following benefits to trainees:

1.   It reverses age-related gene expression.
2.   It increases Brain Derived Neurotrophic Factor (BDNF)

elevations (an important mediator of improving brain functioning), which staves off or reverses age-related cognitive decline and dementia.

3. It increases gut motility, which correlates with muscle mass. One's risk of gastrointestinal cancer inversely correlates with gut motility.

4. It further plays a role in increasing internal organ mass (organ mass also correlates with muscle mass). If you should get in an accident or severely burn yourself, the time you have in the ICU before you die is correlated with organ mass. More muscle gives you more time on the clock.

5. If you were to get in a car accident, the kind of conditioning that strength training gives you may be the difference between three days of whiplash symptoms and a lifetime in a wheelchair (which will be a shortened lifetime).

6. High-intensity training enacts a hormonal cascade that is the antithesis of the metabolic syndrome, thus helping to stave off high blood pressure, elevated cholesterol levels, and obesity.

7. Enhances nitric oxide synthetase: you will have good blood pressure and will never need the little blue pill. You will not need to worry about "being healthy enough for sexual activity."

8. Bone mineral density correlates with muscle mass. Even in osteopenia, strong muscles absorb forces and prevent fractures.

9. Increases your basal metabolism and hormonal profile, which helps to fight obesity.

10. You just look and feel good.

There is even evidence that having more muscle and strength will help to stave off cancer.[2] So the "deal or no deal" question is this: Are you willing to tolerate no more than nine to 12 minutes of high-energy output activity once every seven to 10 days if there was a chance that doing so would result in your becoming stronger, moving better, feeling better, maintaining or improving your health, adding some muscle, and reducing your present level of body fat? Wouldn't that be a "deal" worth taking, particularly when compared to the other health and fitness options that are offered the general public that are long on hype but short on results?

To top it off, resistance training does not require a lot of time out of your weekly schedule, which, as a minimalist in such matters, should broaden its appeal for being the exercise of choice considerably.

I am of course aware that most people have their favorite exercise activity, and I personally would never stand in the way of anybody exercising in the manner that they so choose, but if one truly believes that one's time on this earth is limited and finite, then it follows that one should want to have as much of it available as possible in order to enjoy all that life has to offer. And if one accepts this premise, it further follows that one should spend no more time engaged in exercise than is minimally required to achieve as many of the benefits as possible from what exercise might provide. I would further ask you to consider this—from cardiovascular fitness[3, 4] to muscular strength, to endurance, to flexibility, to the prevention of and rehabilitation from injury, to the relief of mental stress—resistance training can do it all, and it's the only method of exercise that involves all of these components of total fitness within a single method.

The health benefits associated with this one method of exercise are considerable as well, including:

1. Decreased gastrointestinal transit time (reducing the risk of colon cancer)[5]
2. Increased resting metabolic rate[6]
3. Improved glucose metabolism[7]
4. Improved blood-lipid profiles[8, 9]
5. Reduced resting blood pressure[10, 11]
6. Improved bone mineral density[12]
7. Pain and discomfort reduction for those suffering from arthritis[13]
8. Decreased lower back pain[14, 15]
9. Enhanced flexibility[16]
10. Improved maximal aerobic capacity[17]

For those involved in athletics, resistance training can stave off the potential for injury by strengthening joints, muscles, tendons, bones, and ligaments, in addition to augmenting many of the attributes associated with physical performance, such as improving an athlete's endurance, strength, power, speed, and vertical jump.[18] And, as we shall see, all of these benefits can be accomplished with a very minimal time investment.

RESISTANCE TRAINING AND AGE REVERSAL

Perhaps the biggest news to come out of the scientific community is the news that resistance training can actually reverse the aging process. You read that correctly; a study[19] has revealed that resistance training for people 65 and older can actually *reverse* important aging effects in skeletal muscles to the point where they work more like those found in people 40 years younger. The study was supported by the US National Institute of Health and looked at DNA expression in muscle cells of 25 healthy seniors who had undergone resistance training for six months. It concentrated in particular on the cellular mitochondria, the "powerhouses" that fuel activity in cells. They are typically depleted in older people, with many of the genes that affect them turned on or off by age. This depletion results in a loss of muscle mass and many of the mobility restrictions that are often found in seniors. The lead researcher in the study, Dr. Mark Tarnopolsky, said the genetic "fingerprints" of exercising seniors actually shifted from their age-altered state to one more closely resembling those found in young men and women in their mid 20s to 30s. "We improved or reversed to a large extent the gene signature of aging," he said. This reversal was accompanied by a 50 percent improvement in strength among seniors. He went on to state that weight training might remove some of the mitochondria damaged by age-related stresses, replacing them with genetically intact ones. As well, resistance training may turn on genes that have been switched off by age and that offer muscle cells protection from damage. The seniors in the study, who had an average age of 70, had no diseases that affected their mitochondrial function and had never participated in resistance training before.

In addition, although it is tough to top "reversing the aging process" as a benefit, there are even more benefits to resistance training that should be pointed out. Researchers have discovered that many of the degenerative diseases and most of the general weakness that accompanies the aging process are related to a loss of muscle mass and strength. Although a certain amount of strength loss is inevitable, numerous studies—too many to be ignored—have shown that senior adults can maintain and regain muscle mass and strength at any age. Postmenopausal women, older men, and even those well into their nineties have all improved their muscular and skeleton structure and function through relatively simple and brief programs of strength training.

The clinically established results from resistance training are nothing short of remarkable for young and old alike. A study conducted by physiologist Wayne Wescott with seniors to determine the benefits of a brief resistance exercise training program on the body composition, muscle strength, joint flexibility, and functional ability of 19 nonambulatory senior citizens revealed some very encouraging news.

Over a span of 14 weeks, training but twice a week for six minutes a workout, performing one set of each of six different exercises, the senior residents of John Knox Village Campus (which included the Medical Center, Assisted Living, and Independent Living facilities in Orange City, Florida, the average age of which was 88 and a half years) were able to dramatically improve their body composition, muscle strength, joint flexibility, functional capacity, and mobility. Many of the seniors who started the study confined to a wheelchair were able to walk without its aid at the study's conclusion. The 19 subjects who completed the 14-week strength-training program reported that it was a positive experience and planned to continue their exercise sessions. According to the lead trainer, patients liked the challenge of serious strength training and saw much more improvement than when on a program of resistance exercise with light cuff weights. The researchers concluded that in addition to the benefits to our senior population, such programs could be helpful to all ages, and instrumental in reducing health care costs, thereby benefiting society in general.

ONCE A WEEK

In keeping with a minimalist philosophy, an ideal exercise program would be one that takes up as little time as necessary from our busy lives but that still sufficiently stimulates our bodies to produce as many of the positive results listed above that our genetic predispositions will allow. And unlike other forms of exercise that are lower in their ability to output energy and, thus, require longer and more frequently performed bouts to drop the body's energy levels to a degree that is meaningful enough to warrant a positive adaptive change taking place, resistance training exercise can take as little as six to 12 minutes to perform and very satisfactory and sufficient results can be obtained by engaging in it as infrequently as once a week. I will go into greater detail as to why this is so in a later chapter, but for the moment I will point out that a study published in the *Journal of the American Geriatrics Society* in 1999 (47[10]: 1208–14) indicated that the time required for resistance training to stimulate such benefits could be obtained with only one workout a week—and, as we will see, there are more studies that support such a frequency. Indeed, a second comparison of once-weekly strength training in older adults conducted by the Academic Health Care Center of the New York College of Osteopathic Medicine and the Department of Physical Therapy, at the New York Institute of Technology, School of Health Professions, Behavioral and Life Sciences, concluded that one set of exercises performed once weekly to the point of muscle fatigue improved strength. Twice-weekly exercises in the older adult also improved strength.

The interesting thing about strength training once a week is that it not only respects each individual's time and lifestyle (i.e., you don't have to embrace some nebulous concept known in the vernacular as "the fitness lifestyle" in order to be fit and healthy), but such infrequent training is actually a necessity for optimal results to take place.

THE ANTI-AGING PRESCRIPTION

I have touched upon the benefits of resistance training for our senior population, but the importance of this activity for this group of individuals warrants additional consideration. There exist 10 biomarkers of aging:

1. Bone density: Because calcium tends to be lost from the bones when people age, it makes the skeleton weaker, less dense, and more brittle, which typically leads to osteoporosis.
2. Body temperature regulation: The body is supposed to maintain an internal temperature of 98.6 degrees, but as people grow older they tend to lose muscle and the heat that muscle provides, thus

becoming more vulnerable in their body temperature to hot and cold, which often leads to illness—or worse.

3.   Basal metabolic rate: Our rate of energizing or determining how many calories our bodies require to sustain their internal processes declines by 2 percent per decade after the age of 20.

4.   Blood sugar tolerance: The body's ability to use glucose in the bloodstream declines with age, thereby raising the risk for type 2 diabetes, which is one of the fastest growing diseases in the country.

5.   A decline in muscle strength: Older people are less strong because of the gradual deterioration of the muscles and motor nerves, which begins at the age of 30 for most people.

6.   The fat content of the body: Between the ages of 20 and 65, the average person doubles his ratio of fat to muscle. This process is exacerbated by a sedentary lifestyle and overeating. Exercise can often serve to retard appetite and, therefore, when you're not training, you tend to be more hungry—and to eat more often.

7.   Aerobic capacity: By the age of 65 the body's ability to use oxygen efficiently declines by 30 to 40 percent.

8.   Cholesterol and HDL ratios: Around age 50 HDL (or High Density Lipoproteins, the so-called "good" cholesterol that protects the body against heart disease) loses ground to the LDL (or Low Density Lipoproteins, the so-called "bad" cholesterol)—a phenomenon that dramatically increases the risk of heart attack.

9.   A decline in muscle mass: The average North American loses 6.6 pounds of muscle with each decade after young adulthood and the rate of loss increases after the age of 45 (but only if you don't do anything to replace it).

10. Blood pressure: The majority of North Americans show a steady increase of blood pressure with each decade of age.

And the one (and only) activity that has been proven scientifically to positively affect all of these biomarkers of aging indicated above is resistance training. No other activity has proven to even come close.

In case the above weren't enough to convince you to at least consider resistance training as your preferred mode of exercise, the Canadian

Broadcasting Corporation (CBC) reported on a study done in British Columbia that showed that resistance training also served to stave off dementia in older women. It concluded:

> Seniors who lifted weights or did other forms of resistance training slowed their decline to full-blown dementia. A six-month strength training program that targeted women with mild cognitive impairment and who complained of memory problems helped improve their attention, problem-solving and decision-making brain functions—all needed to live independently.[20]

Whether you're young or old, start a resistance training program. It doesn't matter where you start (a gym, your home, etc.)—but start. It is no longer merely an opinion that resistance training is the best form of exercise, but rather a scientifically validated fact. The sooner you employ resistance training as your choice of exercise, your quality of life will increase enormously.

CHAPTER THIRTEEN

THE DᴇLORME AND WATKINS METHOD

L et us suppose that after reading the foregoing you are convinced that you want to begin a resistance training program. Now comes the difficult part for most people—which program should you employ?

There is certainly no shortage of resistance training programs to choose from. But if time is important to you and you would prefer a program with time-tested results, you might be intrigued to learn that despite all of the resistance training programs that have come into the world over the decades, very few (if any) have produced anything close to the results that have been produced by a protocol that was engineered by two medical practitioners over 70 years ago.

The names Thomas DeLorme and Arthur Watkins are unknown to most people, and yet, given how important resistance training has proven to be—assisting with everything from functional ability to reversing the aging process—these two men were truly pioneers in this field. DeLorme and Watkins were both medical doctors and, quite apart from the preventative medicine benefits indicated above, they recognized early on the tremendous rehabilitation benefits afforded by resistance training during their work in helping rehabilitate wounded soldiers during the Second World War.

DeLorme was an orthopedic surgeon by profession who had trained with weights for many years. He knew from his own fitness training experience as well as from his medical training that there was nothing about making an individual stronger that in any way posed a liability to that person's well-being. Indeed, he observed that making an individual stronger actually served as tremendous preventative medicine against that individual becoming infirm in the future. After achieving such remarkable success using resistance exercise in their rehabilitation of soldiers, DeLorme and Watkins published the results of their work in 1951, in a book entitled *Progressive Resistance Exercise: Technic and Medical Application.* It became (and remains well over half a century later) the foundation of all variations of progressive resistance training.

THREE SETS OF TEN

The protocol that Delorme and Watkins found to be most successful was a simple one: three sets of 10 repetitions for each exercise. The sequence moved from lighter to heavier weights with each successive set. As the reader will recall from a previous chapter, warming up a muscle prior to having it perform in a demanding fashion is a good thing. And this protocol, by means of more thoroughly warming up the targeted musculature, serves to prevent injuries to muscles, tendons, ligaments, and joints and also to better prepare the muscles for the final and most demanding set (the "work set") to follow.[1]

The first two of the three sets performed are, in effect, "warm up" sets, with DeLorme and Watkins believing that performing such sets serves to elevate the temperature within a muscle, which will have a positive effect on what they termed "the viscous and elastic properties of the contractile tissue in a manner designed to augment the work done at the same production of energy by accelerating the chemical processes involved. . . . By initial use of small muscle loads and increasing them after each set of 10 repetitions, the muscle is warmed up preparatory to exerting its maximum power for 10 repetitions."

Both doctors also cautioned against making the first two sets too demanding in leading up to the final work set:

The warm-up should not interfere with the performance of 10 repetitions with the 10-Rep Maximum (RM). In other words, if by doing 10 repetitions with the first weight (50 per cent of the 10-RM) and 10 with the second weight (75 per cent of the 10-RM) the patient is too tired to perform the 10 repetitions with the 10-RM, then only five repetitions should be performed in the first two sets, thus leaving the patient fresher for the 10 repetitions with the 10-RM. Another possibility is to omit the middle 10-repetition set (75 per cent of 10-RM), starting then with 10 repetitions with the 50 per cent of the 10-RM and going directly to 10 repetitions with the 10-RM.

Interestingly, they note that the warm-up sets preceding the final set of 10 repetitions actually allow for a better performance on the final set:

> Frequently patients are unable to perform 10 repetitions with the 10-RM if this resistance is applied without preliminary exercise with lighter weights.

I have found in training clients that it is important to get them used to outputting progressively higher amounts of energy (i.e., tapping the Fast-Twitch fibers), and the DeLorme and Watkins method of performing three progressively heavier sets seems to ease the trainee into doing this quite nicely. The first set of 10 repetitions can be considered a warm-up set that uses exclusively Slow-Twitch fibers; the second set, a little heavier, calls upon what's left of the Slow-Twitch fibers as well as bringing some Intermediate-Twitch fibers into play; and the final set, which is also the heaviest, serves to fatigue what's left of the Intermediate-Twitch fibers and brings the Fast-Twitch fibers into play, resulting in a protocol that maximizes fiber involvement and stimulates all of the metabolic processes of the body.

I have found that this protocol works best with three to five multi-joint or compound exercises, but more can be performed in a given workout using the same protocol if one's energy levels are particularly high or if one feels that one didn't quite give all that he or she had to the three or five exercises performed previously.

In terms of selecting a starting resistance to employ, select a weight for each of these exercises that allows for 10 repetitions. If your muscles start to fatigue after five or six repetitions, then the weight you have selected was too heavy. On the other hand, if you can do 20 or 30 repetitions, then the weight is obviously too light. Make the necessary adjustments during your next workout and try to move along steadily from one exercise to the next with a minimal (30 seconds to one minute) rest in between sets and exercises.

So why did DeLorme and Watkins advocate three sets rather than, say, five, six, or more sets per exercise? According to them:

> In the initial publications concerning progressive resistance exercise, 70 to 100 repetitions were advocated, the repetitions being performed in 7 to 10 sets with 10 repetitions per set. Further experience has shown that this figure is too high, and that in most cases a total of 20 to 30 repetitions is far more satisfactory. Fewer repetitions permit exercise with heavier muscle loads, thereby yielding greater and more rapid muscle hypertrophy.

**Note: Although it is not mandatory to have a personal trainer guide you through the exercises that follow, the reader may find it helpful (particularly if you are new to resistance training) to consult with a trainer prior to commencing your resistance training program in order to ensure that proper form is maintained during the performance of the exercises.

MACHINE WORKOUT

LEG PRESS

The Leg Press exercise hits the entire lower body from the waist down with particular emphasis on the glutes, hamstrings, and the quadriceps muscles on the front of the thighs. There is even some rotation around the ankle joint, which serves to involve the calf muscles of the lower leg as well. To begin the exercise, sit down in the Leg Press machine. The seat should be set so that your upper thighs are as perpendicular to the ceiling as possible, with the knees bent so that the shins are bent approximately 90 degrees to the thighs. In other words, one's hips should be flexed slightly more than 90 degrees, and one's knees should be bent as close to 90 degrees as possible. Next, slowly and smoothly push your legs out to a point just short of lock out. We don't want the knees to be locked out, as this creates a loss of muscle involvement when the bones of the lower extremities align. From this position, slowly return to the starting

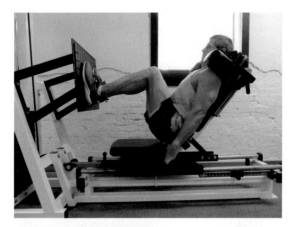

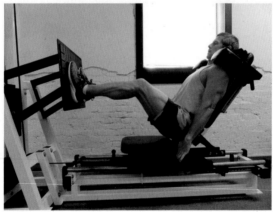

position. Repeat for 10 repetitions. Rest for 30 seconds or so, until your breathing is comfortable. Increase the resistance by approximately 10 percent and repeat the exercise for another set of 10 repetitions. Rest for another 30 seconds. Increase the resistance again by approximately 10 percent and repeat the exercise for a final set of 10 repetitions. Try not to grip the handles on the machine tightly. The body is a closed hydraulic system, and excessive gripping can serve to spike blood pressure levels unnecessarily high.

SEATED ROW

The Seated Row is what is popularly referred to as an upper body "pulling" exercise, targeting the upper back, shoulders, and arm muscles. When performing the seated row, the position of the arms is going to be somewhat predicated on the handgrips of the machine relative to your shoulder width. Ideally, this should be a "natural" position; i.e., you should not deliberately be trying to tuck your elbows in or flare them out, but rather let them ride in the natural plane that they tend to move along. Draw your upper arms back until your hands are just in front of your torso, pause briefly in this position, and then extend your arms back to the starting position, making sure to not simply "drop" the weight in between repetitions but to control it deliberately all the way back and all the way forward. Repeat for 10 repetitions. Rest for 30 seconds or so, until your breathing is comfortable. Increase the resistance by approximately 10 percent and repeat the exercise for another set of 10 repetitions. Rest for another 30 seconds. Increase the resistance again by approximately 10 percent and repeat the exercise for a final set of 10 repetitions.

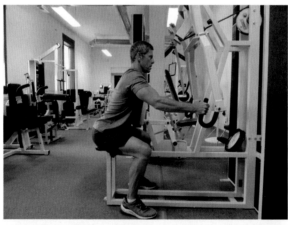

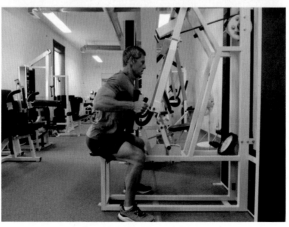

CHEST PRESS

The chest press is an upper body "pushing" exercise, which involves the chest, shoulder, and triceps muscles. The Chest Press exercise is performed the opposite of the Seated Row exercise; i.e., you will be pushing the handles of the machine away from your body as your arms extend. Start the movement with your hands just in front of your chest and press them upward (if you are using a bench press machine that requires you to lie on your back) or forward (if your bench press machine is vertical). Again, don't spend too much time in the locked-out position, as the muscular involvement is minimized when the bones of the arms align in a locked-out position. Now lower the resistance under full muscular control back to the starting position. Repeat for 10 repetitions. Rest for 30 seconds or so, until your breathing is comfortable. Increase the resistance by approximately 10 percent and repeat the exercise for another set of 10 repetitions. Rest for another 30 seconds. Increase the resistance again by approximately 10 percent and repeat the exercise for a final set of 10 repetitions.

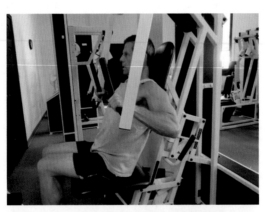

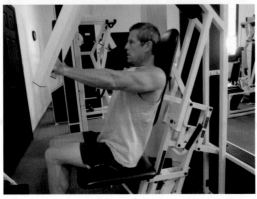

FREE WEIGHT WORKOUT

No. 1: Military Press

Many years ago, Steve Reeves told me that when training he believed it was important to exercise the legs last in a workout. This was largely because when he was competing, the primary form of resistance exercise was barbell and dumbbell training and that if one trained one's legs first, it would weaken the primary means of support for the body and, thus, compromise one's ability to use barbells in movements that required a solid foundation, such as overhead presses. I believe Reeves had a point and, if you are going to train with barbells, then legs should be trained last.

The first exercise performed will be the Military or Overhead Press. This exercise works directly on the triceps and shoulders, but also strongly involves the clavicular portion of the chest, abdominals, and lower back. The triceps are underrated, but they play an important role in throwing and swimming, and they give balance to upper-arm strength. Bend over,

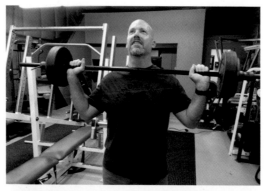

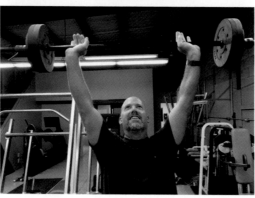

and using an overhand grip, hands about six inches apart, pick up the bar. Your feet should be about shoulder width apart. Stand up with your back straight, or sit straight on a bench. Bring the bar to a position directly over your head; then lower the bar slowly down to your upper chest. When the bar reaches your chest, immediately change direction and press the bar back to the overhead position. Repeat for 10 repetitions. Rest for 30 seconds or so, until your breathing is comfortable. Increase the resistance by approximately 10 percent and repeat the exercise for another set of 10 repetitions. Rest for another 30 seconds. Increase the resistance again by approximately 10 percent and repeat the exercise for a final set of 10 repetitions.

Reminder: Keep your back as straight as you can and your head up. This is not an easy exercise, so don't try to use too much weight at first.

No. 2: Bench Press

Comment: Since the chest and triceps muscles were strongly involved in the Military Press exercise they are already thoroughly warmed up, so the next movement performed will be the Bench Press. Since the chest, shoulders, and triceps are all involved in this exercise you'll be able to handle quite a bit of weight. It takes a certain amount of skill to raise and lower the weight in the proper form and under control, so it may be helpful to practice with a light weight to get the feel of things. If you don't have a weight bench or a suitable substitute, you can do these presses on the floor or on an exercise mat.

Directions: Pick up the bar with an overhand grip, hands about shoulder width apart or a little wider. Bring the bar to your chest as you did for the squat, slowly sit down on the end of the bench, then lower yourself slowly until your back is flat on the bench and your head is resting comfortably. Keep your feet flat on the floor and slightly spread for leverage. Now press the bar straight up from the chest until your elbows are straight and your arms are fully extended. Pause at the top and lower the bar slowly and carefully until it just touches your chest. If you're using a bench, your elbows will be below the line of the bench in the bottom position. If you're on the floor, your elbows will touch the floor, and the bar may not quite touch your chest.

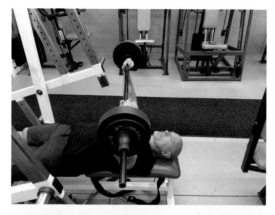

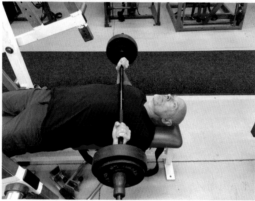

Reminder: Don't sit too close to the edge of the bench unless it is very stable because it might pop up behind you. Keep your buttocks on the bench at all times and try to arch your back slightly.

No. 3: Bent-Over Rows

This exercise works the entire shoulder area—the smaller muscles of the back, the broad latissimus muscles that span the back, the trapezius that supports the neck and shoulders, and the lower back and arms. Stand with your feet comfortably spread apart. Keeping the legs as straight as possible (knees-locked position), bend over at the waist until your back is parallel with the floor. Take the bar in an overhand grip with the hands slightly wider than shoulder width, and bring the bar off the floor a few inches (if you have to bend the knees to pick up the bar, that's perfectly all right). Pull the bar to the chest without moving the upper body. Slowly

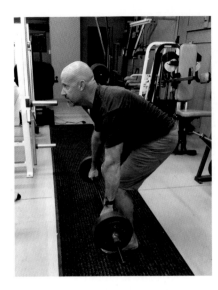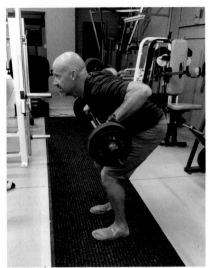

lower the bar back to the starting position. Repeat for 10 repetitions. Rest for 30 seconds or so, until your breathing is comfortable. Increase the resistance by approximately 10 percent and repeat the exercise for another set of 10 repetitions. Rest for another 30 seconds. Increase the resistance again by approximately 10 percent and repeat the exercise for a final set of 10 repetitions.

Reminder: This exercise is for the back primarily, but naturally the arms get some work as well. Don't let gravity take the bar away from the chest; keep the bar under control.

No. 4: Curls

The barbell curl is probably the simplest of the biceps exercises, but it produces quick results. And it's still true that people tend to judge muscularity by the size of the biceps. Bend over and pick up the bar with an underhand grip, hands a little more than shoulder width apart. Stand up and bring the bar up, using your legs and back until the bar is at arm's length in front of you—about mid-thigh. Keeping your feet comfortably spread, curl the bar up until it touches your chest. Make sure your back is straight and your head up throughout the exercise. Pause at the top and slowly lower the bar to the mid-thigh position. Repeat for 10 repetitions. Rest for 30 seconds or so, until your breathing is comfortable. Increase the resistance by approximately 10 percent and repeat the exercise for

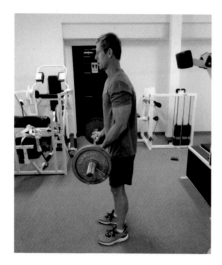 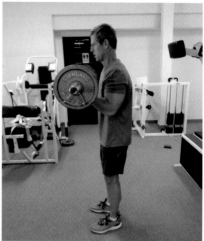

another set of 10 repetitions. Rest for another 30 seconds. Increase the resistance again by approximately 10 percent and repeat the exercise for a final set of 10 repetitions.

Reminder: Try to keep your style and form during the curls. This means holding the shoulders back and using only the arms for leverage and the elbows as pivots. Lower the bar rather than letting it fall back to the starting position.

No. 5: Squats

Squats benefit the legs and the entire back as well, and serve as a good overall stimulus to the body, as they involve most of the large muscles in one movement. Stand with your feet comfortably spread apart. Make sure you have a strong, stable foundation. Bend over, flexing the knees, and grip the bar with an overhand grip, hands a little wider than shoulder width apart. Keep the head up and the back as flat as possible. Using the upper legs and lower back, bring the bar straight up in a plane parallel with the body. Keep the arms straight until the bar passes the knees, then begin to bend the elbows and prepare to tuck them under the bar as it reaches chest level. Get underneath the bar and bring it to rest on the upper chest, just under the chin. Next, press the bar upward and then lower it behind your head so that it rests comfortably across the shoulders and the base of the neck. Adjust the weight and your stance until you're steady and well balanced, then squat as if sitting until your thighs are

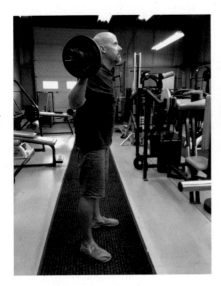 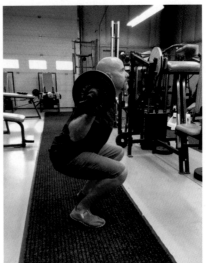

just below parallel. The feet should be flat on the floor at all times. Pause at the bottom to eliminate momentum that can be created by bouncing, and then slowly raise yourself back to the starting position. It's important to remember that this is not an arm exercise. Use only the legs and back. Keep your head up at all times by focusing on the point where the ceiling meets the wall. If you're having any trouble with balance, try putting a small board under your heels. Repeat for 10 repetitions. Rest for 30 seconds or so, until your breathing is comfortable. Increase the resistance by approximately 10 percent and repeat the exercise for another set of 10 repetitions. Rest for another 30 seconds. Increase the resistance again by approximately 10 percent and repeat the exercise for a final set of 10 repetitions.

OPTIONAL FREE WEIGHT EXERCISES

No. 6: Deadlift

The movement involved in the deadlift provides exercise for the lower back, strengthening the muscles and relieving tension at the same time. But this is really a good whole-body exercise as well; it serves to prevent lower back problems, which are the most common medical complaints among athletes and the general public as well. Take the same starting position as you did for the bent-over rows. Bend over at the waist, flexing

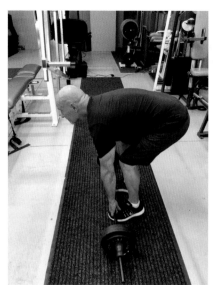
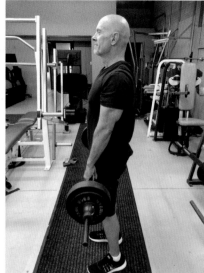

the knees just a little, and grip the bar with an overhand grip, hands a little wider than shoulder width apart. Straighten the legs and lift the bar off the floor a few inches. Keep your back as straight as you can, and keep your head up. Now, lifting with your legs, stand erect with the bar. Keep arms straight and shoulders back in the standing position. Bend over and lower the weight until it touches the floor. Repeat for 10 repetitions. Rest for 30 seconds or so, until your breathing is comfortable. Increase the resistance by approximately 10 percent and repeat the exercise for another set of 10 repetitions. Rest for another 30 seconds. Increase the resistance again by approximately 10 percent and repeat the exercise for a final set of 10 repetitions.

Reminder: For the most benefit, be sure to exaggerate the shoulder movement when you reach the standing position by thrusting the shoulders back and the chest out. If you need to bend your knees more than suggested, go ahead and do so. You'll eventually be able to do the lift in proper form.

No. 7: Toe Raises
Muscles: Lower leg
You can use a barbell placed across the top of your back (as in Squats) for this exercise. This is the best and simplest exercise for strengthening the calf muscles.

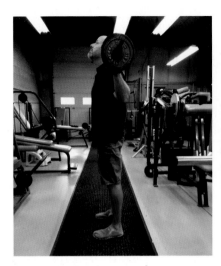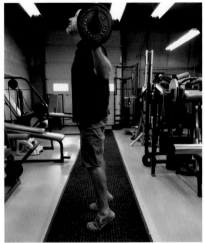

Stand with your back straight, your head up, and the barbell resting across the top of your shoulders. Lock your knees and raise up as
high as you can on your toes. Hold at the top for a count of two and
then slowly lower your heels back to the floor. If you want to increase
the stretching motion, stand with your toes on a small block of wood,
letting your heels touch the floor. Repeat for 10 repetitions. Rest for 30
seconds or so, until your breathing is comfortable. Increase the resistance by approximately 10 percent and repeat the exercise for another
set of 10 repetitions. Rest for another 30 seconds. Increase the resistance again by approximately 10 percent and repeat the exercise for a
final set of 10 repetitions.

Reminder: Whether you use a block of wood or not, balance can be
a problem with toe raises. With a little practice, however, you'll quickly
get the hang of it.

No. 8: Bent-Leg Sit-Ups

Lie flat on your back on the floor and flex your knees until your feet
also are flat on the floor. Place your hands across your chest. Next, curl
your body up from the waist until your torso almost touches your thighs,
and then pause for a count of two before lowering yourself back to the
starting position. This is one exercise where you don't have to start with
three sets of 10 repetitions, as the abdominal muscles receive a lot of indi-
rect work from the preceding free weight exercises. Instead, start with 10

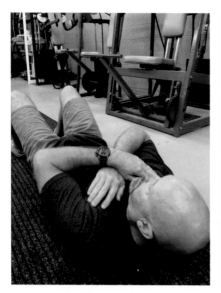 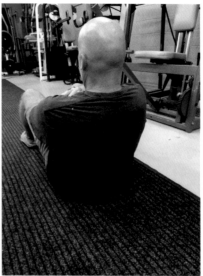

repetitions and add one sit-up every workout. When you can perform 25 repetitions, you can increase the intensity of the exercise by holding a light weight across your chest.

Reminder: This is a stomach exercise, so if you feel any strain in your legs or back, increase your concentration and make sure the abdomen is getting the work. Don't bounce up from the floor because it will be momentum doing the work, not you.

MORE EXERCISES ARE NOT NECESSARY

As the reader will have noted, the above exercises work the major musculature of the entire body, and most of the minor ones as well—neck, upper back, shoulders, lower back, chest, biceps, triceps, buttocks, front thighs, hamstrings, calves, and abdomen. I would suggest that you stick with either one of the programs outlined above for at least 12 workouts; that's three-months' worth of work if you maintain the schedule of one workout per week. At that point you will want to consider some changes to your program. Recall that the C.E.P. is constantly at play.

I can't claim anything original in this program; it's simply a tried-and-true result-producing workout that can be performed in any commercial gym or home with any basic barbell set. And while other workout programs may make claims about being "more efficient," "stimulating greater growth," and being "state of the art," these are, for the most part, simply marketing claims. The amount of muscle one can build is governed by certain biological and hormonal influences, and most of us will have tapped out our potential for building muscle mass within the first three years of our training. What the DeLorme and Watkins method offers is a "bird in the hand" when it comes to proven muscle-building benefits. The other protocols, while perhaps effective, simply don't have the proven track record to be anything more (at this juncture anyway) than "two in the bush" (to follow through with our analogy). Even the renowned bodybuilding champion and movie star Steve Reeves only used three sets for each of his exercises when in peak form, and he told me once that for people over the age of 50 who were looking to get into shape or maintain their shape and condition that they should do no more than three sets—total—per muscle group. As the program outlined above works many muscle groups simultaneously, three exercises performed for three sets each in total are all that's required.

In conclusion, then, the DeLorme and Watkins protocol has been time proven in its effectiveness. And while I'll introduce some alternative training programs to you in the next chapters, for beginners it's always preferable to go with a sure thing—and the DeLorme and Watkins method is as close to that as has ever been offered in resistance training.

CHAPTER FOURTEEN

THE MAX PYRAMID PROTOCOL

Ever since acquiring a suntan became fashionable, people have been going out into the direct sunlight for hours at a time, several days a week, in order to increase the melanin production in their bodies and acquire as deep a tan as possible. Over the years, the process of acquiring a tan in such a fashion has been revealed to have its drawbacks, as almost from the get-go some people were overdosing on their exposure to direct sunlight. Blisters, burning, and premature wrinkles were not uncommon side effects from such a practice. And while people long knew that "something" about exposure to direct sunlight was responsible for the tan they sought, they weren't certain as to what exactly this "something" was. However, they quickly learned, often to their cost, that there was also something about repeated exposure to direct sunlight that also produced a negative and decidedly opposite effect to the one that they were seeking.

These observations resulted in a general consensus that while exposure to direct sunlight contained the stimulus that moved one further along the path to the tan he or she sought, it only did so up to a very definite point. After this point was reached, more time in the sun stimulated the production of nothing positive. In fact, it did terrible things, particularly when it was discovered that quite apart from the burning and the blisters was the very real threat of skin cancer (melanoma). Then there was the fact that only a small percentage of the population seemed to be able to acquire a deep, dark tan; the rest fell into a spectrum that turned their skin color anywhere from pink to light brown to beet red. Along the way, it was discovered that there was even a segment of the population that could not tolerate any direct sunlight exposure at all. And so it seemed that there was a strong genetic component attached to the issue of tolerance to direct sunlight and the acquisition of a suntan.

When cancer was identified as being a very real threat, sunlight was held up to scientific scrutiny and was discovered to have many components, among them being ambient light, radiant heat, and UV radiation. Due to the fact that tanning was not going away despite its implications for negative health, this new information was examined critically by those who cared to do so. Ambient light and radiant heat were discarded almost immediately as not being study-worthy, as it was obvious that neither contributed anything to the tanning stimulus. UV radiation, however, was another matter entirely. And once the researchers had isolated UV radiation as being the agent that served as the necessary stimulus to the body to produce a suntan, a new industry came into being. Suntan lamps were created and proved popular with the general public and, as more was being discovered about the tanning potency of UV radiation, eventually a "tanning bed" was created that would allow those who desired a tan to obtain one with as little as one 10-minute UV radiation session a week—as opposed to the multiple hours per week that used to be spent by most people who sought to acquire a tan.

The above represents an organic process of stimulus and response involving the human body. A very similar situation exists with the body's response to exercise. Similar to our suntanning analogy, it wasn't that long ago that a similar situation existed in the health and fitness world. For the longest time nobody knew exactly what it was about demanding muscular activity that made our bodies stronger and healthier compared to those who did not partake in such activities. Those who were sedentary tended toward weakness, obesity, and ill health, whereas it was observed that those who routinely performed demanding muscular work grew stronger and maintained their health for a much longer period of time. Soon, those seeking to become healthier and stronger began to engage in demanding muscular work on a regular basis. They jogged, they ran marathons, they stretched, they lifted weights, they swam, they cycled, and many did these activities as often as they could. Again, nobody at the time really knew what it was about demanding muscular activity that resulted in our bodies producing the desired effect, only that something about this activity seemed to result in this adaptation.

However, as with the ambient light and radiant heat in the sunlight example, it was discovered over time that there were elements within muscular activity that were decidedly negative to our health and strength aspirations. There were, it was observed, significant wear and tear factors and huge force issues associated with muscular activity that, over time, could become chronic and ultimately do us more harm than good. And, as with the vast genetic variation that exists in regard to the tanning response, there likewise were those people who never seemed to get as strong or healthy as others did by engaging in the activity of demanding muscular work, so obviously there was a genetic factor at play here as well. Fortunately, over the years, it was discovered that the stimulus within demanding muscular work that served to make us stronger and healthier was the outputting of large amounts of stored energy from within muscle tissue taken to the point where the muscles' energy output dropped to a level that made the continuation of the activity being performed very difficult. With this in mind, i.e., that the stimulus required is a momentary weakening of our muscles (an emptying of their fuel supply), it then became possible to examine whether it was possible to isolate and impose this stimulus in a manner that would mitigate (if not eradicate) the negative factors so indicated.

Knowing that wear and tear is a result of muscular motion, and that irrespective of the supplemental exercise we might opt to engage in we still must expose ourselves to some degree of wear and tear through necessary daily activity, the question becomes is there at least a means by which we can minimize this wear and tear during our exercise sessions? And if the stimulus we are seeking is an emptying of energy out of our muscles, is there a point in the normal range of motion of our limbs that sees the muscles outputting more energy than at other points in their range of motion? The answer to both questions, it would seem, is yes.

The protocol that I am about to present in this chapter has proven so successful with regard to the previous points indicated that it has unofficially become the "house protocol" at my facility. It takes into account lessons learned and studies conducted with my previous motionless exercise protocols such as *Static Contraction Training* (McGraw-Hill, 1998), *Max Contraction Training* (McGraw-Hill, 2003), and *Advanced Max Contraction Training* (McGraw-Hill, 2006), as well as insights gleaned from dialogues with individuals who have made a thorough study of the biomechanics of exercise and how it relates to muscular structures. In particular, the work of Bill DeSimone, author of *Moment Arm Exercise* and *Congruent Exercise*, has helped guide me, as have Kinesiology professors at several Canadian universities. According to DeSimone, the position of maximum moment arm is the one point in a given muscle's range of motion where the muscular structures are outputting energy at their maximum:

> The most challenging position of an exercise is the mechanical sticking point, or a maximum moment arm. With free weights, it is where the weight is at the farthest horizontal distance from the joint. . . . With cam-based machines, it's where the chain or cable comes off the largest radius of the cam. With plate-loaded, leverage machines, it is again where the weight is at the greatest horizontal distance from the axis of the loading arm. . . .[1]

In essence, maximum moment arm is where your leverage is the worst, resulting in your muscles having to work harder by recruiting fibers more aggressively to sustain or generate a contraction. By contrast, when, for example, your legs or arms are in a locked-out position (such as when one's legs are fully extended in a Leg Press or one's arms are fully extended in an Overhead or Bench Press), your leverage may be optimal in such a position but the moment arm is minimal, and, thus, your muscle fiber involvement will be reduced to some degree (depending upon the load employed and the degree of involvement of the bones for support). The hold point in Max Pyramid training (the point where you hold the resistance statically) should be the weakest point in your range of motion owing to the disadvantageous leverage. However, this doesn't mean that the fiber stimulation isn't maximal. A muscle may be loaded in different points (with loads that correspond to the strength of the lever system) of the range of motion and a sequential fiber recruitment will still take place until all available fibers have been recruited and fatigued. However, as I'll point out shortly, a heavy load isn't necessary to recruit all available muscle fibers if you use leverage to your (dis)advantage. And this is a desirable thing, as another negative component in exercise is the potential for injury owing to increases in force, and as force is defined as "mass x acceleration," anything we can do to diminish the weight or load (mass) you are having your muscles work against will therefore diminish the forces that come back to your joints and connective tissues. If you remain in this one position where your muscles are working their hardest (i.e., outputting the greatest amount of energy), you will have diminished acceleration to "zero," thus removing the other component of the force equation.

It stands to reason that you will be outputting energy to a much greater degree if, for the sake of illustration, you complete a Leg Press exercise and are unable to sustain a contraction against 60 pounds of resistance rather than if you complete a Leg Press exercise and are unable to sustain a contraction against 150 pounds of resistance. Thus, the fatigue (or effective energy output) from exercising in the position of maximum moment arm (the position where your strength is not expressed greatly but that is the most difficult) is actually greater.

TIME AND LOAD

The protocol, for wont of a better name, I've labeled "Max Pyramid," as it involves engaging your muscles at the point of maximum moment arm, and it is to be performed in a pyramiding fashion. In fact, it involves the trainee ascending to the "top" or apex of the pyramid (load wise) and then descending back down to the pyramid's base. As there are no repetitions to count with this protocol I use what is called a "Time Under Load" method of measuring performance, whereby one counts the seconds of a given set, in addition to recording the resistance employed. The clock is started as soon as the selected resistance leaves the weight stack and is stopped when it returns to the weight stack on the final set. Several sets are employed throughout the duration of this one "set" and this is done as much for psychological reasons as physiological ones. If one were to only use one set (and this is not to say that one shouldn't do this from time to time) of sustaining a contraction in the position of maximum moment arm and then "wait out" the sequential recruitment and fatiguing that ensues over a time span of, say, 60 to 90 seconds, it can be very challenging mentally, as the trainee knows that the discomfort from the lactic acid burn (as the higher-order fibers are recruited) is only going to get worse, and it will require an unusually high degree of self-motivation to stay the course when that course is so unpleasant.

I have found that starting at a very light (i.e., nonthreatening) weight and then building up over the course of, say, three minutes via a series of progressive sets, ensures that the muscles trained are thoroughly warmed up prior to hitting your top weight (a la the DeLorme and Watkins protocol), while also allowing the client to more subtly bring the lactic acid burn from a simmer to a boil without getting too anxious or wanting to terminate the set prematurely. Our purpose with this protocol is to achieve a "sequential recruitment" of motor units, from the lower order (Slow Twitch) fibers all the way up to the highest order (Fast Twitch) fibers, including all of the fibers in between (Intermediate Twitch) as best we can in an uninterrupted manner. Our objective in refining the stimulus of demanding muscular work, however, is not to demonstrate our strength (i.e., the lifting of the heaviest weight possible), but rather to stimulate our muscles to become stronger. More importantly, in the bigger picture, our objective is to stimulate our metabolism, such as our aerobic and anaerobic systems and to achieve a "glycogen dump" out of our muscles, to allow the circulating glucose a place to go, thus giving us a little more latitude in our diet and also maintaining a stable insulin sensitivity on the surface of our muscle cells. This allows for enduring health benefits, apart from the cosmetics of bigger, shapelier muscles.

It's not uncommon for me to blindfold my clients when they are first using this protocol, as I want to disabuse them of the notion that they are "lifting" weights. Instead, I have them focus on *contracting against resistance*. This may seem inconsequential, but it is a distinction that eliminates ancillary muscular involvement and shifting in the seat or fighting for a leverage advantage during the performance of an exercise. From my perspective, "how much weight" they lift is not important; I'm training my clients to become stronger, not to become performance artists in strength shows. How much weight they lift is irrelevant to my purpose, which is to momentarily weaken their muscles. To this end, it is far more important to see how "little weight" they can finish a set with, as this is a solid measurement of how momentarily weakened their muscles are. If, for instance, a trainee can maximally lift 100 pounds and I give him or her 90 pounds of resistance, he or she will terminate his exercise at the moment his or her strength dips below 90 pounds, resulting in a temporary weakening of the muscles being trained by somewhere between 10 and 11 percent. By contrast, if I can get that same trainee to be unable to move 40 pounds, then I will have momentarily weakened his or her muscles somewhere in the neighborhood of 60 to 61 percent. This results in a much greater degree of momentary fatigue being imposed and, thus, a much stronger signal being sent to his body to become stronger. As Dr. Doug McGuff has pointed out, "All your body knows at the end of [such] a set is that *it couldn't move*. Mobility is a very well preserved biological function, as if you can't move then you can't get food and you can't avoid becoming food." Coming as we do from a hunter-gatherer past, this momentary weakening of muscle is taken very seriously by your body, and this sets the stage for it to make an adaptive response by getting stronger and storing more bio-chemicals (such as glycogen, the glucose polymer that is stored in muscles) as a defensive reaction. Remember that the majority of a muscle's volume is water, and water bonds to glycogen at a ratio of three grams per gram, so the more glycogen you can output from your muscles, the more your body will put back in and (given the bio-chemistry of your body) the bigger your muscles will get. While there are other elements that also result in a muscle growing larger, such as a thickening of the actual muscle tissue as a result of minor damage, the momentary fatigue model subsumes most (if not all) of the effective stimulus elements.

THE MAX PYRAMID PROTOCOL

Now to the protocol itself. I deliberately start the trainee out with a weight that is nonthreatening to him or her. This serves the double benefit of creating a progressive warmup of sorts, and not unduly involving certain bodily defensive mechanisms such as the golgi tendon organs, which can terminate a contraction before full fiber involvement takes place. I emphasize that the trainee "contract" against the resistance—rather than "lift," "thrust" or simply "move" the resistance, as the former enhances focus, develops a stronger neuromuscular connection between the mind and the muscles being trained, and also loads the muscles more effectively. The trainee then moves his or her limbs into a position of maximum moment arm for the major muscle group(s) he or she is training and remains in this position for 20 seconds. The 20-second count is performed to set the recruitment/fatigue process in motion and to ensure the arrival of positive failure prior to heavy weights being employed (thus reducing the force coming back to his or her body). However, I've found that by limiting the trainee's focus and discomfort to a series of 20-second intervals, I can achieve an effective muscular loading and sequential recruitment of fibers and, knowing that there is a miniscule "break" forthcoming after 20 seconds, the trainee is more disposed to continue on with the process of soldiering up (and down) the mountain, so to speak.

Once the first 20-second count is complete, the trainee slowly returns the resistance under control to the weight stack, whereupon the trainer immediately moves the pin down one notch on the weight stack and the trainee is once again instructed to "contract" his or her muscles against the resistance. This procedure is continued until the load and fatigue combine to the point where the trainee either cannot lift the weight from the stack or cannot sustain his or her contraction against the resistance for a full 20 seconds. At this point we reverse direction and—in the exact same fashion—proceed to have the trainee work his or her way back up the weight stack until he eventually returns to the load level he started with. These "contractions" (this series of static holds) can be likened to the "repetitions" of a conventional set, with each successive contraction, like each successive repetition, serving to recruit and fatigue more and more motor units over the span of time of a conventional set until all available motor units (and motor unit types) have been recruited and fatigued out. An example of a Max Pyramid set on the Leg Press, then, might look something like this:

1st contraction: 80 lbs x 20 seconds

2nd contraction: 90 lbs x 20 seconds

3rd contraction: 100 lbs x 20 seconds

4th contraction: 110 lbs x 20 seconds

5th contraction: 100 lbs x 20 seconds

6th contraction: 90 lbs x 20 seconds

7th contraction: 80 lbs x 20 seconds

Allowing for the additional time required to raise and lower the weight (albeit only an inch or two) into position and the time required to pull out and reinsert the pin into a weight stack, the total time of this process would be in the neighborhood of two minutes and 40 seconds (give or take). The total time for a process such as this will vary depending upon the predominant fiber type that an individual possesses in a given muscle group, with trainees that are Fast-Twitch dominant having a shorter time and those that are Slow-Twitch dominant requiring a longer time.

After working his or her way back up the stack to his starting weight, the trainee will note that the same resistance that felt like nothing when he or she began the exercise now feels particularly challenging. And, after maxing out on his or her way down the stack, as he or she works his or her way back up and the weights get progressively lighter, the trainee will be able to more effectively control his contractions, thus keeping the load squarely on the targeted musculature as it progressively weakens. The trainee's respiration will now be palpable as his cardiovascular system kicks in to process the lactic acid out of his muscles (which, you will recall, it does by back-engineering it to pyruvate and processing it through the aerobic system). This protocol is best performed on specialized resistance training machines, but it can also be adapted for use with bodyweight-only and barbell exercises.

MAX PYRAMID PROGRAM (USING EXERCISE MACHINES)

When using resistance-training machines, the distance the trainee should move the weight to begin each exercise is minimal, perhaps one inch on an exercise such as the Leg Press. This places the muscle group being targeted in its worst possible leverage position, which means that muscular involvement will be at its highest since there are no structures other than muscular that are contributing to the movement or to the "holding" of the resistance. The distance the trainee will move his limbs to get to the position of maximum moment arm will vary depending upon the length of the involved levers (limb length) and the exercise he is performing. Since we typically only perform a "Big 3" or a variant thereof, here are the approximate "hold" points for these three exercises:

1. LEG PRESS: The Leg Press machine should be preset so that when the trainee is seated in the machine his or her thighs are perpendicular to the ceiling. In other words, one's hips should be flexed slightly more than 90 degrees, and one's knees should be bent as close to 90 degrees as possible. At this point the trainee should slowly and smoothly push his or her legs out slightly until the weights are approximately one inch off the stack.

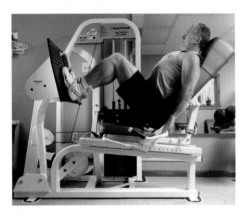

2. LAT PULLDOWN: From a position where your arms are fully extended above your head, slowly pull them down until your upper arms are at a 90-degree angle to your body.

3. OVERHEAD PRESS: Take hold of the handle bars on the Overhead Press machine and slowly push your arms upward until your upper arms are at a 90-degree angle to your body and the weights are approximately one to three inches off the weight stack.

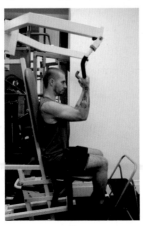
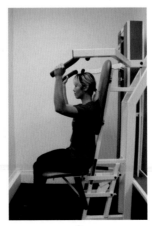

2   3

The Leg Press and Overhead Press positions are approximate, and will still require the trainee to locate his or her own "sweet spot" where he or she feels his or her leverage to be the worst and the loading of his or her muscles the most. The Lat Pulldown can be made into an incredibly effective exercise that works almost every muscle in the upper body by incorporating the following six elements into its performance:

1. The torso should be at a 90-degree angle to the legs.
2. Draw the humerus down until it is 90 degrees from the torso (that's the hold point).
3. Hyper-supinate the wrists so that your palms are facing east and west (or as close to that as you can).
4. Draw the elbows together until they touch in front of you while keeping your upper arms at a 90-degree angle.
5. "Crunch" your abdominals by compressing your trunk downward (not by bending forward or by lowering your upper arms out of the 90-degree position).
6. Remember to "contract" into and out of the "Max Moment Arm" (again, for wont of a better term) position—don't think about "moving" or "lifting" weight, but rather "contracting" against the resistance.

MAX PYRAMID PROGRAM (USING BODYWEIGHT)

The Max Pyramid Program using your bodyweight will make use of leverage changes throughout a movement's range of motion. As you are stronger in certain points in the range of motion of certain postures than you are at other points, you will be using moment arm principles to vary the resistance for you as you move up and down throughout the range of motion.

1. Wall Squats: Place your back against a wall and bend your legs slightly. Sustain this position for 20 seconds. Now lower yourself about four inches and sustain this position for another 20 seconds. Lower yourself again until your legs are just above being parallel with the floor and sustain this position for an additional

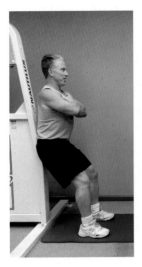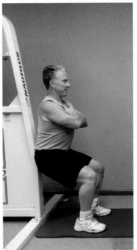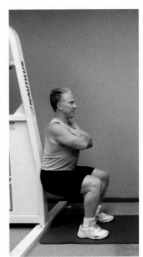

20 seconds. Lower yourself until your legs are at a 90-degree angle to your torso and sustain this position for 20 seconds. At this point, repeat the process but in reverse; i.e., by moving yourself up with each 20-second interval until you are back to the position in which you started the exercise. Tip: If you find you can perform this entire sequence of sliding up and down the wall without much burn in your legs, then add weight to the movement by holding a light dumbbell in each hand.

2. PUSH-UPS: Start the exercise just shy of the arms-locked straight arm (or top) position of a push-up. Sustain this position for 20 seconds. Lower yourself a couple of inches and sustain this position for another 20 seconds. Lower yourself another two inches or so and sustain this position for 20 seconds. Lower yourself just shy of your upper arms being parallel to the floor and sustain this position for 20 seconds. Then lower yourself until your upper arms are parallel with the floor and sustain this position (maximum moment arm) for another 20 seconds. Now reverse the process, pushing yourself back up one position at a time and sustaining each position for 20 seconds until you reach the position from which you started the exercise. Tip: If you find it too difficult to do a conventional push-up, start out by keeping your knees on the ground during the exercise. As you grow stronger,

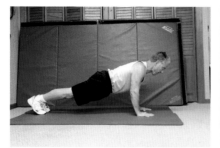
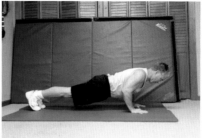

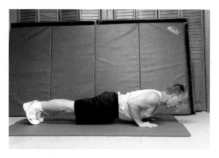

you will be able to perform this exercise in the conventional fashion.

3. PULL-UP BETWEEN CHAIRS: You will need a bar or strong broomstick of sorts. Lie on your back on the floor between two chairs and place the bar between them. Taking hold of the bar with a palms-up (facing away from you) grip, pull yourself up two inches or so until your upper back is just off the floor. Sustain this position for 20 seconds. Then pull yourself up a little bit higher and sustain this position for another 20 seconds. Pull yourself up another two inches and sustain this position for 20

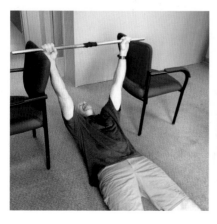
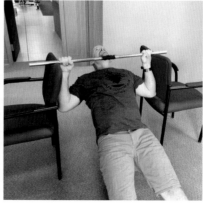

seconds. Now pull yourself up as high as you can and sustain this position for 20 seconds. At this point reverse the process and begin to slowly lower yourself, stopping at each of the points in the range of motion that you paused at on the way up. Sustain each of these positions for 20 seconds until you return to the position from which you started the exercise.

MAX PYRAMID PROGRAM (USING A BARBELL)

The Max Pyramid Barbell Program will make use of similar leverage principles as were employed in the bodyweight program, so that the actual resistance or weight on the barbell will remain the same but it will feel heavier or lighter as you move into maximum and minimum moment arm positions.

1. BARBELL SQUAT: Place a light barbell across the top of your shoulders and bend your knees slightly. Sustain this position for 20 seconds. Lower yourself about five inches and sustain this position for 20 seconds. Lower yourself another five inches and sustain this position for another 20 seconds. Lower yourself again, this time just shy of your upper legs being parallel with the floor and sustain this position for 20 seconds. Now lower yourself until your thighs are parallel to the floor and hold this position for 20 seconds. Now reverse this series of holds at five-inch

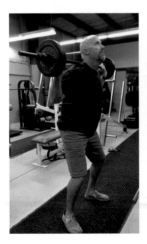
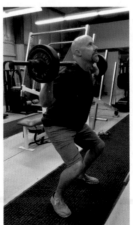
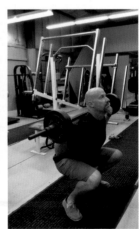

intervals, pausing for 20 seconds at each stage until you have returned to the starting position.

2. BENT-OVER ROW: Bending forward at the waist, take hold of a moderately weighted barbell. Pull the barbell upward about three inches toward your chest. Hold this contraction for 20 seconds. Pull the barbell upward another three inches and pause for 20 seconds again. Pull the barbell upward another three inches and sustain this contraction for 20 seconds. Now pull the barbell up until it almost touches your chest and sustain this contraction for 20 seconds. At this point, lower the barbell three inches and sustain this position for 20 seconds and repeat this process until you have returned to the starting position.

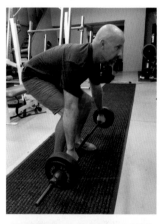 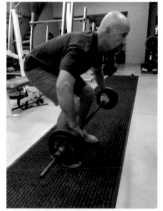

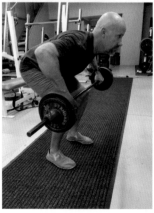 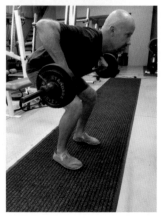

3. BENCH PRESS: Lying back upon a bench, grasp hold of a bar-
    bell and extend it to arm's length above your chest. Bend your
    arms slightly (perhaps two inches) and sustain this position for
    20 seconds. Lower the bar another two inches and hold this posi-
    tion for another 20 seconds. Lower the bar again until your upper
    arms are almost parallel to the floor and sustain this position for
    20 seconds. Now lower the bar until your arms are parallel with
    the floor (the position of maximum moment arm) and sustain
    this position for 20 seconds. Now reverse the sequence and hold
    each position for 20 seconds as you press the barbell back to the
    starting position.

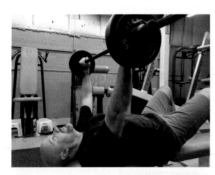 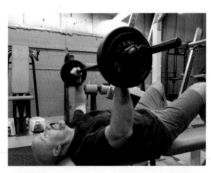

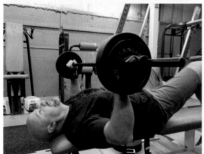 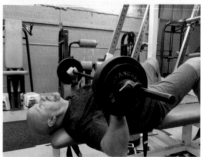

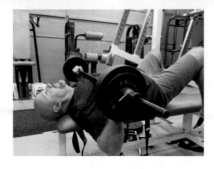

What I personally like about this protocol is that when you engage your muscles in the position of maximum moment arm a modest resistance is all that is required. The need for heavier and heavier weights is negated by the fact that you can, in effect, make a lighter weight seem like a much heavier weight to your muscles. This is a good thing not only from a practical standpoint but also for safety purposes, as it keeps the forces that you will be exposed to quite low. Newton's Second Law reveals that when you push out against 200 pounds of resistance, 200 pounds of resistance pushes back at you, so using progressively (and perhaps needlessly) heavier weights on a barbell or on a machine can create a growing "force" problem for the joints and connective tissues of trainees as they grow stronger. Fortunately, by employing the moment arm principle, your muscles can be thoroughly stimulated to grow stronger while the forces they are exposed to in the training necessary to achieve this result can be kept quite low.

There is a long-held belief in strength training circles that one simply must lift the heaviest weights one is capable of if one wants to build stronger muscles. However, while it may be true that a stronger muscle can lift a heavier resistance, lifting a heavier resistance is not the only way to build a stronger muscle. A study conducted by McMaster University in Hamilton, Ontario (Canada), examined the effect of heavy weights (training load) on the muscle growth process and came to the conclusion that as long as one worked his or her muscles to the point of muscular failure; i.e., the point in a set when another repetition becomes impossible, then it made no difference at all whether the resistance used is heavy (in this instance 90 percent of the subject's One Repetition Maximum weight) or light (30 percent of the subject's One Repetition Maximum Weight).[2] As long as the muscle group being trained was trained to the point of no longer being able to contract, that was sufficient stimulus to the body to make that muscle bigger and stronger. And when the principle of maximum moment arm is brought into play, you can effectively bring about a sequential recruitment of motor units throughout a muscle until all of its available motor units have been stimulated (from Slow-Twitch through Intermediate-Twitch to Fast-Twitch). And as maximum moment arm is the point where the targeted muscle group is outputting the maximal amount of energy, there exists no reason to compromise the potency of this stimulus by moving out of this position (hence the "hold" at this point).

For most experienced trainees, two such exercises in a given workout have proven to be sufficient. Beginners to strength training might be able to recover from more exercises performed in Max Pyramid fashion, but recall that when you are tapping Fast-Twitch motor units you will be tapping "Fight or Flight" fibers. Consequently, there is a corresponding release of the stress hormone cortisol when one does this, which means that the muscles now must not only recover the energy resources that they had expended during the workout (and where necessary repair any micro-trauma that might have taken place), but also deal with processing the cortisol—both of which are biological processes that require time. Consequently, one can very easily set up a situation whereby one will be spending many more days below baseline than above it, which clearly should not be the goal of one's training.

CHAPTER FIFTEEN

ONE AND DONE!

From my present-day vantage point I note that most training programs and protocols can serve to stimulate the production of health and strength benefits. There has been no shortage of excellent physiques, stronger muscles, and better health demonstrated by people who have trained with but one set of an exercise carried to a point where another repetition in good form was impossible (as my old friend Mike Mentzer advocated), three sets of 10 repetitions per muscle group (as DeLorme and Watkins advised), and various permutations of the above. Similarly, I have noted people achieve success training three times per week or training only once a week, and using protocols that emphasized negative-only repetitions (whereby the trainee doesn't even lift the weight but simply focuses on the lowering of it after someone else lifts it into position for him), partial repetitions, full-range repetitions—the list goes on and on. So in terms of the "stimulus" side of the ledger, every form of resistance exercise would appear to "work" to some degree to help us realize our physiological potential. However, our individual physiological potential varies tremendously and, more importantly, is a fixed genetic trait; i.e., it cannot be transcended irrespective of the training protocol employed.

So if we are to grant parity to all resistance training protocols, we can pick whichever one we like. However, if safety is a factor—and it ought to be, as it will determine how long you can continue to train (i.e., you can't train if you're constantly injured)—it becomes apparent that not all exercise protocols will receive a check mark in the "safety" side of the ledger and many produce excessive wear and tear and force en route to stimulating whatever positive adaptations one might have the genetics to obtain. Moreover, we also know that however well designed our exercise program may be, it will eventually cease to be productive once the C.E.P. kicks in to stem the outflow of energy from our muscular system. And so our exercise program must change periodically in order to bump our progress balloon back up into the air again. However, we don't want to engage in random physical activity in our quest to perform high-energy output activity. We want our exercise sessions to minimize wear and tear and force factors and still accomplish the desired objective. With that in mind I would like to introduce in this chapter a protocol called One And Done! And, as its name suggests, it involves the performance of one repetition, but this one repetition must be performed very slowly.

Conventional repetitions are typically performed rather rapidly as the trainee has it in his or her mind that he or she has to reach a certain number, such as 10. Consequently, little attention is paid to the first several repetitions of the set, as reaching that final repetition number is the goal. The result is that the typical trainee will move into and out of the position of maximum moment arm quite quickly during the performance of his or her set, thus only partaking intermittently of the high-energy output benefit afforded from this position. However, if instead one performs but one repetition and performs this repetition very slowly, making sure to spend considerable time in the position of maximum moment arm, some interesting things happen. For one, fiber recruitment and energy output will be increased considerably while moving through the position of leverage disadvantage where the muscles, rather than the bones, are the major contributor to supporting the load. Indeed, by moving so slowly through the position of maximum moment arm, by the time one reaches a position of leverage advantage, whereby the load is decreased to some degree, that decrease is just enough to allow one to complete the repetition (it actually feels as though the load has not been decreased at all). Making an effort to recruit all three classes of muscle fiber in one repetition is not easy, but is much easier on your joints than performing two, three, or 10 repetitions. Even the skeptic who believes that the wear and tear differential between, say, a 10-repetition set and a one-repetition set is minimal, must concede that a 10-repetition set presents 10 times the opening and closing of the hinge joints in the elbows, and, thus, 10 times the effective rate of wear and tear, that a one-repetition set does. In addition, the One and Done! method is much easier on one's psyche as well, as one only has to endure the fire of the lactic acid burn once—and then it's over—rather than having to endure it repeatedly over several sets.

THE PYRAMID OF FIRE

As unpleasant as it unquestionably is, the lactic acid burn is a necessary part of the high-energy output process. You can liken any muscle on the body to a pyramid; i.e., the fibers comprising the base of the pyramid are Slow-Twitch; there's plenty of them, but they are not very powerful (which is why we need a lot of them to do our various day-to-day tasks). Not being particularly powerful, they emit a miniscule exhaust (which we perceive as a burning sensation). Proceeding on to the middle of the pyramid we encounter the Intermediate-Twitch fibers. There are not as many of these as there are Slow-Twitch fibers, but they must do the same workload that their slower twitching but more populous cousins do. Consequently, they are more powerful engines and emit a more power-ful exhaust than do Slow-Twitch fibers. Again, we perceive the exhaust from these fibers as a burning sensation (lactic acid) and, the higher up the pyramid we ascend, the hotter this burning sensation becomes. And just as the apex of the pyramid is the narrowest section, we typically have fewer Fast-Twitch fibers than we do Intermediate and Slow-Twitch, with the result that these fewer fibers again must do the same workload that required more of the lower order fibers to accomplish. Additionally, while there are fewer of these fibers, they possess the same power as the bulk of the lower order fibers and, being more powerful, the exhaust from these fibers is considerable! But as long as you are aware of an increase in the burn you are experiencing from your muscles, you know that you are successfully ascending to the top of the pyramid in terms of muscle fiber involvement. This can easily be done with one slow, controlled repetition. Moreover, it is important to keep in mind that you cannot stimulate into growth fibers that are not involved (recruited) in an exercise, so if you're not experiencing the burn, you are not involving and stimulating all of the fibers that you should be.

When performing this one slow repetition, you do not want the movement to degenerate into a series of stops and starts, but rather to proceed with a smooth continuous contraction until you have reached full contraction of the limbs you are training. Once you've reached this point, you will then slowly and smoothly reverse direction and lower the resistance back to the position at which you started. If you have done this properly, you will be unable to complete (or even initiate) a second repetition. In other words, you will have called into play and exhausted all three classes of muscle fibers. The process is akin to pedaling a bike up a very steep hill; the closer you get to the summit, the greater the burn in your legs until you can no longer pedal any further. However, unlike bicycling, it won't require hundreds of revolutions of the pedals (which is simply more wear and tear) to fatigue your fibers to this point. Instead, it takes but one repetition.

WEIGHT

As we've seen, lifting very heavy weights isn't necessary for training purposes. For the One and Done! method, simply select a modest weight that you can fully control within the weakest position of a given muscle group's range of motion. When you are in your weakest position, you are in the position of maximum moment arm, that one position where your muscle tissue will be working its hardest. When load and position combine at this point in the range of motion it is like an accelerant has been poured on the muscle fiber recruitment process, as the bones are not helping to support the load during the lifting and lowering. As a result, as you exit the position of maximum moment arm to one of a more favorable leverage position, you do so considerably weaker than you were heading into it, thereby creating a variable resistance effect that tends to track with your force output capabilities throughout the range of motion.

If one employs a heavy weight in one's exercises, the tendency will be to move quicker through the position of maximum moment arm (where you can recruit fibers more readily) and into a position where the bones contribute to the bearing of the load (rather than just the muscles), with the result that you will hit muscular failure prematurely (i.e., as soon as you fatigue sufficiently so that the weight is too heavy in the position of maximum moment arm). Consequently, you will not have stimulated as many fibers as possible. While developing this protocol I tried adding more weight and reducing the time that the muscles were under load from upwards of three minutes down to 90 seconds and even 60 seconds, but, speaking for myself, I found that my muscles were more thoroughly stimulated if I used a lighter weight and really took my time in the range of motion where the exercise feels the most difficult. The total time a given set lasted would vary for me, as there was a greater energy-output from leg exercise that saw the duration last between three and four minutes, while for my upper body exercises it was a range of two to three minutes. This may be just me, however, so feel free to experiment to find out what Time Under Load produces the best effect for you (in fact, varying your time under load for each exercise might actually result in a better overall stimulus being imposed on your muscles). However, with an eye toward reducing force and wear and tear issues, with a more modest weight and a slightly longer Time Under Load (TUL), I feel as though I am involving a greater amount of fibers and fatiguing them even more thoroughly, as evidenced by the fact that it takes me longer to regain the strength necessary to walk when I hit the wall with a lighter load on the Leg Press than it does when I do so with a heavier load. What's fascinating is that the One & Done! protocol accomplishes this deep fatigue and stimulation of the muscles in a manner that reduces both mass (load) and acceleration (speed), which, again, are the two components by which "force" is defined. In addition, it dramatically reduces the amount of wear and tear one's joints are exposed to almost exponentially, as it is harder to imagine anything less in volume than one repetition when it comes to exercising a group of muscles.

To date, I have had best results in performing the One and Done! protocol with a three-exercise workout, typically a Leg Press, a Pulldown, and an Overhead Press if you have access to a commercial gymnasium with resistance training machines; a Deep Knee Bend, Push-Up, and Pull-Up between two chairs if you are just using bodyweight; and a Squat, Overhead Press, and Curl if you are using a barbell set. However, it can just as easily be performed with any exercise, even in a workout that consists of more exercises (although I'm sure the trainee would be exhausted after the first three exercises, rendering the remaining exercises somewhat superfluous). You could also experiment and change the exercises on an alternating basis (i.e., use the Leg Press, Pulldown, and Overhead Press one week, and a Squat or Leg Extension/Leg Curl combination, together with a Chest Press and Seated Row the next week). The protocol works equally as well with isolation movements.

EMPLOYING THE PROTOCOL

Depending upon which equipment you have available, perform one set each of the three exercises listed in the categories below.

BODYWEIGHT	BARBELL	EXERCISE MACHINE
Push-up	Standing Press	Chest Press
Deep Knee Bends	Squat	Leg Press
Pull-Up (between chairs)	Curl	Seated Row

BODYWEIGHT PROGRAM

1. PUSH-UP: Lie down on the floor on your stomach. Place your hands just below your shoulders. Keeping your body tight and with only the toes of your feet and the palms of your hands touching the ground, slowly begin to press your body upward until your arms are fully locked out. Lower from this position back to the starting position. Tips: Initiate the pressing motion very slowly and when you reach the top, arms locked position, do not linger there for long as that is the one position in the exercise where the bones (when in the arms locked position) take

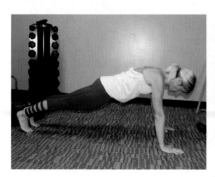
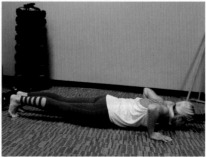

the majority of the load rather than the muscles. Once you reach the top position, slowly begin to lower yourself back to the starting position. Move as slowly as you can on both the upward and downward portion of the press. When you reach the bottom position, attempt to perform a second repetition. You should be unable to move upward. If you find that you can, you performed your previous repetition too quickly. Attempt the second repetition, but make it a mental point to slow down the speed of movement the next time you perform this exercise.

2. DEEP KNEE BEND: From a standing straight position, descend as low as you comfortably can (for some people they will be able to almost touch their buttocks to their heels; for others simply getting close to parallel will suffice). From this lowered position, slowly begin to contract your thigh muscles and, using leg strength only, press yourself back up to a standing position. Lower yourself back down to the starting position. Tip: As with the push-up, don't linger too long in the top position, as the bones in the legs—rather than the muscles—will be bearing the brunt of the resistance when the legs are straight. Slowly lower yourself back to your starting position. Attempt a second repetition. If you cannot complete it, then your speed was just right. If you can, then attempt to reduce your speed even more the next time around.

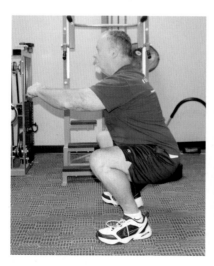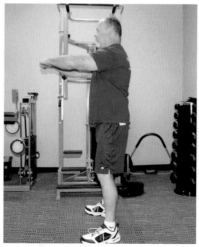

3. PULL-UP (BETWEEN CHAIRS): You will need two chairs and a broomstick handle or long piece of doweling to serve as a bar in order to perform this exercise. Place two chairs on the floor with the backs of the chairs facing each other. The space between the two chairs should be such that you can lie down between them with room on either side. Place the bar across both chairs so that it resembles a chinning bar. Grasping hold of the bar with a shoulder-width grip, lower yourself and extend your legs so that they are in front of your body. From a fully extended position

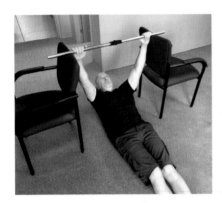 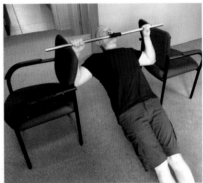

where you are hanging onto the bar, slowly contract the muscles in your arms and upper back, making sure to keep your body straight, and begin to pull yourself up toward the bar. When you reach the top of your ascent, slowly reverse direction and lower yourself under control back to the starting position. Tip: With this exercise you will not have the problem of the bones supporting the resistance, so simply rise up and lower yourself under muscular control. When you have returned to the start position, attempt a second repetition. If you moved slowly enough, a second repetition should be impossible.

BARBELL PROGRAM

1. STANDING PRESS: Pick up a barbell from the floor and lift it up so that it is resting across your upper chest with your palms facing forward. Slowly begin to press the bar upward as slowly

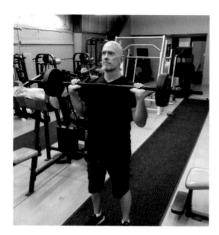
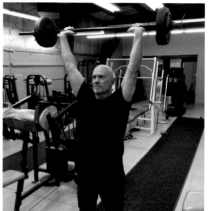

as you can until you reach a straight-arm position. As the bones will assume some of the load in this position, don't linger here; instead, reverse direction and slowly lower the bar back to your upper chest. Tip: Don't allow your back to sway when you are pressing. Instead, keep your back ramrod straight and let your arms and shoulders do the work. Attempt a second repetition once you have returned the bar to the starting position. If you were moving slowly enough, a second repetition will not be possible.

2. CURL: Stand erect with a shoulder-width grip on the barbell and your palms facing front. Your arms should be fully extended so that the barbell is directly in front of your thighs. Now slowly lift, or curl, the barbell up to shoulder height, solely using the muscles of the upper arm by bending the elbows. From this fully

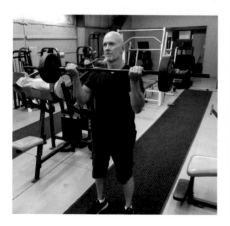
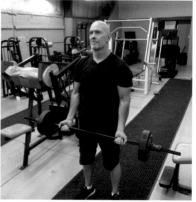

contracted position, slowly lower the resistance back to the fully extended or starting position. Tip: Remember to let only the upper arms do the work during this movement. Fight the tendency to let additional muscle groups come into play by swinging the body or shrugging the shoulders to add momentum to the movement.

3. SQUAT: Stand erect with a barbell across your shoulders and take a deep breath. Now, with your lungs full, bend your knees and lower your body until you are in a full squat position; you should be slightly below a 90-degree angle to your shins. As soon as you reach the bottom position, begin to slowly press yourself back up. Tip: Again, do not linger long in the legs-locked position. Instead, slowly lower yourself back to the starting position

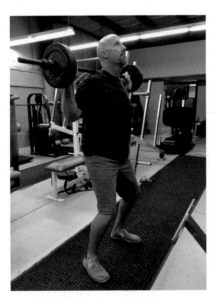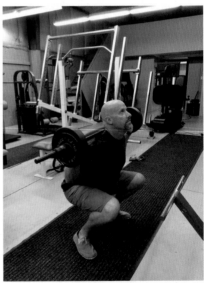

and attempt a second repetition, which should not be possible. Keep your back straight and your head up at all times. If you feel uncomfortable with the bar across your back you can always perform what is commonly called a "Hack Squat," which requires that you hold the bar at arm's length behind you (so that it is just below your buttocks). Bend your knees until the barbell plates touch (or almost touch) the floor, and then begin your ascent from this position.

EXERCISE MACHINES

1. CHEST PRESS: The Chest Press involves the triceps muscles on the back of the upper arm to a great extent, in addition to the deltoid musculature that surrounds the shoulder joint. The pectoral muscles (chest muscles), both pectoralis major and pectoralis minor, are also strongly stimulated by the performance of this exercise. When performing the chest press, you will be pushing the handles of the machine away from your body while simultaneously pulling the humerus toward the midline of your body as your arms extend. Start the movement with the plane of the palms at the front of the armpit. It is important that you neither tuck nor flair the arms excessively; they should be kept

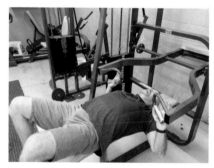 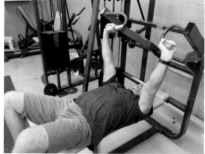

at a 45-degree angle if you're holding the handles appropriately to start, and then you simply press your arms forward smoothly and stop just short of lockout, so that the muscle stays loaded and you're not resting on a bone-on-bone tower with your elbows locked. Lower the resistance slowly and under control. Tip: While you want to achieve a full range of motion in this exercise, it is not necessary or desirable to lower your arms as far down as possible, as doing so will only strain the shoulder capsule and add tension to the biceps tendon at the humeral head.

This is not necessary to thoroughly load the chest, shoulder, and triceps muscles.

2. LEG PRESS: The Leg Press exercise hits the entire lower body from the waist down, with particular emphasis on the hip and buttock musculature. The leg press also strongly involves the hamstring musculature on the back of the thighs, the quadriceps musculature located on the front of the thighs, and to some extent there is also rotation around the ankle joint, which serves to recruit and load the gastrocnemius (or "calf") muscles of the lower leg. The leg press machine should be preset so that when the trainee is seated in the machine in the flexed or tucked position, his or her thighs are perpendicular to the ceiling. In other words, one's hips should be flexed slightly more than 90 degrees, and one's knees should be bent as close to 90 degrees as possible. At this point slowly and smoothly push your legs out to a point

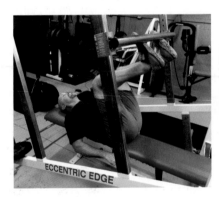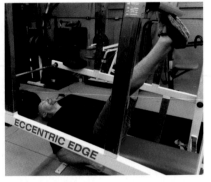

just short of lock-out. Tip: You don't want the legs to be locked out, as this creates a loss of muscle tension during the bone-on-bone tower. From this position, perform a very slow transition or reverse of direction, with the legs now bending until they have returned to the starting position. The movement, inclusive of directional transitions, should be performed in a fluid, smooth circular motion.

3. SEATED ROW: The Seated Row involves the latissimus dorsi muscles, the rhomboid musculature (located between the

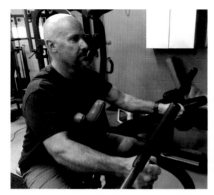 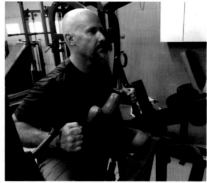

shoulder blades that serve to draw them together), and the spinal extensor muscles that run from the base of your sacrum to the back of your head. Those will be involved as a secondary component from doing this, as well as all the muscles of the flexor side of the forearm that flex your wrist, as well as the biceps and brachioradialas muscle that bend your arm at the elbow joint. When performing the Seated Row, let your arms move as they naturally would in line with your hands, wrists, and shoulders. Starting from an arms-stretched position, slowly contract your arm muscles and begin to draw the handles toward you. When you have drawn your arms back as far as you can, slowly change direction and return the handles to the starting position. Tip: Don't allow your arms to stretch too far forward during this exercise, as doing so will transfer the load from the superficial larger muscles to the deep muscles that bind the shoulder joint (which are not as capable of handling a heavier load as the superficial muscles are).

One of my clients used this protocol exclusively and over a period of six weeks (and in conjunction with a switch to a calorie-reduced diet) dropped the better part of 30 pounds of fat. Moreover, when I tested his body composition in the BodPod machine, I discovered that he had gained six pounds of muscle during this same period. While this may not produce the same results in all trainees, it is at least evidence that the "stimulus" side of the ledger is well represented with this protocol (particularly given that my client was then 53 years old and no stranger to intense muscular work) and, again, the wear and tear and force from such a workout is as miniscule as it can possibly be.

All of my clients (and particularly the ones who have suffered joint problems from years of athletics) that have used the One and Done! protocol have reported how much they like it. They like the fact that they feel as if they've worked their muscles as thoroughly as they have with other high-intensity protocols (and in some instances much more thoroughly) and yet they don't feel beaten up or sore during their non-workout days. I've also found that the learning curve for trainees is very quick with One and Done!, compared to other protocols I have used with my clients in the past. In terms of recovery, working out but once a week appears to be optimal.

ONCE A WEEK—AND DONE!

I have indicated earlier that full recovery and adaptation (i.e., an increase in strength) occurs during the rest period that falls in between workouts, and that this process can occur with a workout that is performed as little as once a week. Many readers will be wondering, *How can this be? How can one workout session a week be enough exercise?* To better understand the answers to these questions it behooves us to look at the science literature to see what actually happens to our bodies as a result of a high-energy output exercise session. According to the medical literature, the more intensely the muscles are made to contract, the more damage or micro trauma that takes place at the cellular level.[1, 4, 5, 7, 9, 10] Consequently, the greater the intensity of the workout, the longer must be the time frame that follows to allow for the repair and growth of the tissues that have been stimulated by the workout. It is this process of repair and growth that makes the muscle fibers bigger and stronger.[2, 9] A high-energy output workout causes some degree of damage to muscle fibers, and during the 24 hours that follow such a workout, inflammation will set in, during which white blood cells (neutrophils) will be increased and be mobilized to the site of the injury.[1, 6, 9] It is during these first 24 hours that enzymes will be produced that serve to break down and metabolize damaged tissue (lysosomes), which adds further to the inflammatory process.[3, 6, 8, 9, 10] For the next several days additional cells that serve to synthesize other chemicals in response to inflammation (macrophages) will act to assist the lysosomes, one of which is PGE2, a cell that is believed to make nerves within muscles more sensitive to pain (which explains to some degree the perception of soreness that one experiences after a workout).[1, 2, 3, 4, 5, 6, 7, 9, 10] This inflammatory response brings some additional damage to the muscles and can continue for several days after the workout.[1, 6, 7, 9] It is only after these inflammatory responses have run their course, signs of tissue remodeling (building of muscle) will then be observed.[4, 7, 9] The muscle fibers build back to their pre-workout size and then, if further time is allowed, they will build up to a level that was greater than it was prior to the workout. The length of time for this entire process to complete itself is dependent upon the intensity of the workout performed and the corresponding damage to the muscle fibers[2, 4, 5, 10] but typically it will fall in the neighborhood of five days (on the quick side of things) to upwards of six weeks.[1–10]

While the above represents a microscopic view of what happens as a result of a single bout of demanding muscular exercise, there have been other studies that looked at the issue of exercise frequency macroscopically, examining the effects of training different groups of people (from senior citizens to younger subjects) with one, two, or more workouts per week. Here is what the science literature has to say on the subject:

In a study conducted by Graves et al., 50 men and women who were accustomed to strength training were divided into three groups and had their training frequencies dialed back from their customary twice or three times a week to once or twice a week. A control group, which didn't train at all, lost 70 percent of the strength they had at the beginning of the 12-week study, but those who reduced their frequency (even to once a week) lost nothing at all.[11] In another study involving strengthening exercises for the lower back, 112 subjects were tested with a variety of frequencies (from three workouts per week to one workout every two weeks). Interestingly, all frequencies resulted in strength increases and the results were essentially the same whether the subjects trained once, twice, or three times per week. Moreover, the data was suggestive of a situation arising of diminishing returns with more frequent training, as the group that trained but once every two weeks gained an average of 26 percent in lower back strength (which is a very respectable return on one's time and energy investment), whereas the group that trained three times a week only gained an average of 14 percent more—but from six workouts as opposed to one workout every two weeks.[12]

Evidence appeared in 1996 that baseball players were able to maintain their strength with one workout per week during the pre-season.[13] In a 1999 study involving senior citizens (aged 65 to 79), a once-weekly strength training session was again shown to be sufficient to improve both strength and neuromuscular performance in older adults.[14] And even for experienced trainees, a lower frequency of training has been shown to produce very effective results. In a study involving recreational weight trainers (who thus had grown accustomed to the rigors of progressive resistance exercise), a group was split in half, with one half training three days per week and the other training once per week utilizing a protocol of employing only one set per exercise (and a total of three exercises) taken to a point where another repetition could not be performed through a full range of motion. At the end of the protocol the group that trained three times a week experienced a greater improvement in their One Rep Max (the amount of weight that a subject can lift one time), but, surprisingly, the group that trained only one day a week produced 62 percent of the One Rep Max that the three times per week group did—while only training two-thirds less.[15]

In a study involving 18 older adults (seven women and 11 men, aged 65 to 79) that were split into two groups (one training once a week and the other training twice a week), the researchers discovered no difference in terms of the rate of strength gain either group experienced, despite one of the groups training twice as much (or 100 percent more in this instance) as the other group.[16] In a study conducted in 2007 to determine the effect on Leg Press strength in two groups of untrained women who were made to perform the Leg Press exercise either once or twice a week, the researchers concluded that the strength gains were essentially the same.[17]

The once-a-week workout is not an aberration; rather it pays attention to the absolutely necessary component of rest and recovery in the body's process of adaptation. Rest is necessary to allow for the full benefit of an exercise session to be produced and, more importantly, in the bigger picture, the rest days in between workout sessions allow the trainee the opportunity to spend more time above baseline so that he or she can make use of the increased strength, energy, and health that his or her high-energy output workouts have stimulated before tearing it down again with another workout.

CHAPTER SIXTEEN

THE FUTURE OF EXERCISE

It's pointless denying it; we live in a computer age. We use our laptops, desktops, and iPads constantly, and our smartphones are as much a part of our selves these days as the hands that hold them. We answer our email, book reservations, obtain our reading material, and are constantly researching things—from used cars to self-help methods—through our portable technology. It was only a matter of time (and some would lament that it is long past time) that technology finally entered the field of exercise. Although we understand the principles (minimal wear and tear, low force, high-energy output, etc.) that are necessary to bring exercise into the 21st century, until recently we were forced to do our best to apply them while using 20th-century equipment. Yet don't misunderstand me—20th-century equipment will most certainly do the job and, given that almost all of the results that one can obtain from exercise are genetically determined and that these tools have long been proven adequate to bring forth such results, there hasn't existed much need to reinvent the wheel in this instance. However, while our results from exercise may not change, the amount of time we need to spend engaged in pursuing them is changing rapidly.

As great a tool for the purpose of exercise as a barbell can be, the invention of certain types of resistance training machines represented an evolution to the application of resistance training to muscles, as the machines reduced the risk for injury and allowed us a safer means to train in a high-energy output manner, which meant that the time required to devote to our workouts was necessarily diminished (as high-energy output exercise and long bouts of exercise are mutually exclusive). This was all to the good. However, the introduction of cams, pulleys, and levers into our training apparatus meant that the amount of weight that was selected for us to be used to train our muscles was often not the actual weight that our muscles were working against. As a result, while progress could be measured on such equipment, its measurement was of necessity imprecise, which from a scientific standpoint represented anything but an evolution. Our muscles produce force in varying degrees as they move throughout their respective ranges of motion, and seldom is this force expressed in convenient chunks of 10-pound increments, such as one might find comprising a weight stack on a resistance-training machine. At the end of the day, apparatus such as barbells and machines only provided us with a gross measurement of the force output of our muscles; i.e., once our strength dipped below the amount of weight on a barbell or weight stack, we could no longer move the resistance, and the exercise ended—but we never knew precisely how far our strength actually dipped. Was it 2 percent? 5 percent? 15 percent? 40 percent?—or some other value in between? It has always been impossible to say. However, technology in resistance exercise has finally entered the digital age, allowing us to know exactly how much strength we are losing during an exercise session (and even during a particular set of a given exercise)—and how much strength (measured in force output) we are gaining as a result of our high-energy-output exercise sessions. In this respect, exercise equipment has—finally—made the move into the 21st century.

Spearheading this advance is the innovative team of Jim Colles, Ryan Guzman, Randy Rindfleisch, and Ariel Huskins at Outstrip Equipment. They have created a force gauge technology that measures precisely how much force is produced by our muscles during every moment of every repetition of exercise we perform and, in keeping with our minimalist approach, Outstrip has manufactured a machine that works every major muscle group in the body and measures the precise amount of force that one's muscles produce. Moreover, it measures this force output on the fly, so the trainee can actually see the inroading or momentary weakening taking place—and to what degree—as it occurs in real time. The equipment that makes use of this technology, called Outstrip, further allows one to output maximum energy safely as there are no bars that can be dropped, no vacuuming of plates on a weight stack that could suddenly drop and, thus, change the counter force requirements dramatically, and no way for a trainee to ever be exposed to more load or force than the trainee's muscles can safely accommodate. The data that is produced during the workout can also be uploaded to a smartphone or a flash drive, thus allowing the trainee to take his or her "workout chart" home with him or her in order to review the results.

Such data is hugely significant, as it allows one to assess one's rate of progress and, should progress arrest at some point, a quick analysis of this data should provide at least a suggestion to the trainee as to what the cause might have been. For example, did he or she recently change his or her diet? Did he or she add supplemental exercises into his weekly routine that collectively had made a deeper inroad into his or her energy reserves and that now requires either more recovery days to compensate for, or that he or she needs to remove from his or her weekly programs because their addition was taking him or her in the wrong direction? One can also now precisely assess whether adding more recovery days in between one's training sessions allows one to make better or worse progress.

The Outstrip machine that I use at my facility is called the Solus, and it allows the trainee to perform a "Big 3" workout routine, consisting of a Leg Press (a lower body pressing movement), a Seated Row (or upper body pulling movement) and a Seated Chest Press (or upper body pressing movement). Once the client gets into this machine he or she doesn't get out until all three movements are performed and the workout is over. The total time of most clients' workouts on this machine is about six minutes, owing to the fact that each repetition performed is so much more draining on the energy reserves within one's muscles than is a repetition performed on more conventional equipment. And as both the number of repetitions per set and the sets per workout

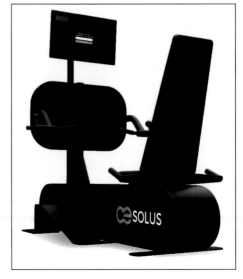

have been reduced of necessity while working out on such a machine, so, too, has the wear and tear factor of exercise, which is a huge step in the right direction.

Part of the reason for the Solus's ability to more efficiently drain one's energy stores is the fact that it allows the trainee to put forth a maximal effort in both the lifting (positive) and lowering (negative) components of every repetition performed. One's negative strength—i.e., one's ability to lower a given resistance under control—has long been known to be significantly (some have put the figure at 40 percent) greater than one's ability to lift a given resistance. So, for example, if you can pull 100 pounds toward you in a Seated Row exercise, you can lower under control approximately 140 pounds. With most exercises the amount of weight you lift is the amount of weight you lower. And given that you cannot lift 40 percent more weight than your maximal concentric or positive ability, then the amount of weight you lift that is optimal for your concentric contractions will be 40 percent lighter for the eccentric or lowering portion of your repetition, which affords you a bit of a rest when you lower the resistance and prepare for your next repetition. Consequently, conventional gravity-based exercise equipment can be said to represent a two steps forward, one step back approach to inroading or fatiguing one's working muscles. Eventually one's muscles will fatigue to a meaningful degree, but after utilizing the Solus it becomes obvious that more conventional apparatus simply requires one to train for a longer period of time in order to fatigue a working muscle, making it obvious that such apparatus—while effective—are less efficient.

By comparison, both portions of the repetition performed on an Solus machine are (or can be) maximally adapted to whatever a trainee's existing strength happens to be on this equipment, making for a very direct line from starting strength to finishing strength with no backward steps or rest periods in between. Consequently, you can achieve in four to five repetitions the same degree of fatigue that would otherwise take you several minutes (with Max Pyramid or One and Done!), or that would require three sets of 10 repetitions (with DeLorme and Watkins) to achieve. For those seeking a more efficient (and thus even more minimalist) approach to exercise, this machine represents just such an innovation.

Unlike most exercise equipment manufacturers, who simply look for a good idea that has proven popular (such as treadmills) and then look for a way to manufacture them less expensively and distribute them more widely, the folks at Outstrip, rather impressively, were driven solely by their passion for actually creating a better, safer, and more thorough way to exercise. I can vouch for this because my gym is a virtual catalogue of team member Randy Rindfleisch's various mental forays into attempting to build a better exercise machine over the years. He started with leverage machines, then adapted a strain gauge to build into his equipment to test torque during Max Contraction (isometric) exercise, and then applied the strain gauge to a motorized pulley in order to allow for dynamic movement that could be performed more safely and that could likewise be measured. His teammates then designed the machine and worked constantly on refining the technology within it until it came to result in the Solus, which is simply the latest evolution of their desire in this regard. Who knows? In five years Outstrip may have refined this application yet again. Interestingly, the Outstrip team has recently been in talks with the lead physiologist at NASA, which has long had to grapple with the physiologic problems (bone demineralization and muscle atrophy) that occur in a weightless or reduced gravity environment. It simply isn't practical (for obvious reasons) to bring a heavy barbell set or circuit of resistance training machines into a spacecraft and then launch it into outer space. The Outstrip concept of a resistance-training machine without a weight stack is, therefore, of considerable interest to them. I can only smile when I think of Mike Mentzer's words to me regarding NASA and exercise, and how impressed he would have been with the Solus in this regard.

I recognize that this technology is rare at the moment and mention it here only to alert the reader to its existence. If you have the opportunity to exercise on one of the Outstrip machines by all means do so, but if such technology is not yet available where you train presently the protocols and equipment indicated previously will work very effectively.

MAX CONTRACTION

Another great protocol to employ on the Solus is that of Max Contraction. In Max Contraction training on the Solus, you select three positions in a given exercise's range of motion—near full extension, the midpoint, and bottom—then you contract maximally in each of these positions for 30 seconds. Take a 15-second rest in between each maximal contraction. I have found that the Chest Press, Seated Row, and Leg Press are perfect for this protocol on this machine. Moreover, the computer retains the data from your previous workout so that you can compare your performances to see if you are tracking upward. It is a great protocol for people who may have sore knees, elbows, or shoulders, as it allows them to have a thorough workout without placing their limbs in a position that will cause pain. Plus, since there is no motion involved, there are no wear and tear forces to worry about. Just remember to breathe continuously, as you would if you were running or performing any other type of demanding muscular activity, and to keep the non-involved muscles (such as the neck) as relaxed as possible.

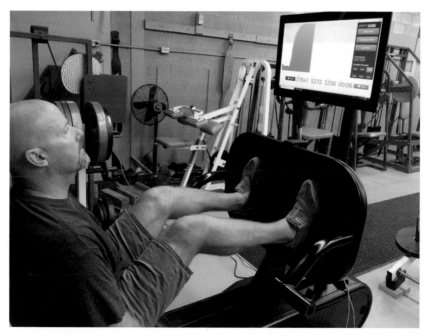

Performing the Max Contraction Leg Press Exercise on the Solus

TRAINING ON THE SOLUS

While there is no shortage of protocols that you can use on this machine (Max Contraction, negative-only, positive-only, hyper reps, Superslow,

DeLorme & Watkins, Max Pyramid, Max Contraction, etc.), I have been really impressed by how demanding it makes the One-And-Done! Protocol. There is literally "zero" rest time during both the positive and negative excursions, making one all-out repetition all that is required to thoroughly stimulate the muscles involved in the Leg Press, Seated Row, and Chest Press exercises. I put the setting on 15 and have my clients start each movement in the position of maximum moment arm and then begin their positive repetition. The total time for a One-And-Done! set can vary, but I have found that one minute on the positive excursion and one minute on the negative excursion will give any trainee all the stimulation that he or she desires. Three exercises that work the whole body, then, can be completed in a total of six minutes. That represents a huge evolution in exercise in terms of reducing wear and tear and maximizing muscle stimulation!

CHAPTER SEVENTEEN

NUTRITION AND FAT LOSS

I must confess at this point that, as a general principle, I do not usually speak on the topic of nutrition unless I'm really pressed to do so. Nutrition has become such a contentious issue over the last several decades, with many people clinging to certain dietary beliefs as if they were sacraments delivered from a higher power, that you almost take your life in your hands whenever you discuss the subject.

These various dietary beliefs are almost as numerous as the people that cling to them, with each belief having its supporters and detractors. Simple logic tells us that if we are looking for an "ultimate truth" in such matters they can't all be right—and yet each group can point to specific examples of successful fat loss within each of their camps that are the direct result of their nutritional practices.

By way of example, witness the low-to-zero carbohydrate proponents who proclaim that calories mean nothing and that carbohydrates (particularly refined carbohydrates) are the villains that are responsible for all of our society's health and obesity issues. The China Study group, by contrast, maintains that carbohydrates in the form of vegetables are the best thing in the world we could eat, and that meat (protein and fat) and dairy products such as milk and cheese are the real culprits of which to be wary. Both of these sides argue for the reduction or elimination of certain macronutrients in one's diet and the sole (or predominant) consumption of another macronutrient. Then there is a group that believes that the secret to great health is to be found in the ratio of macronutrients consumed to one another. To someone who has never looked into nutritional science very thoroughly (or at all), such conflicting opinions can be incredibly confusing.

Adding to the confusion about nutrition is the fact that, like most other factors in human existence, there is a large role that genetics would appear to play in our ability to store (and lose) body fat. Indeed, there is now scientific evidence that some people can eat the same food as others, but have completely different reactions to it in terms of body fat storage. Differences in height, existing fat levels, liver size, and stress hormone levels such as cortisol can each influence the energy utilized to maintain the body's metabolic operation by as much as 600 calories a day.[1] There is even evidence that trillions of microscopic bacteria within our intestines can digest some of the tough or fibrous matter that our stomachs are unable to break down and thereby release a torrent of additional calories in the process. But even these microbes vary in their ability to do this between individuals. So all of this serves to further muddy the waters of nutrition and makes exactitude in matters of diet a bit of a moving target. With all of this conflicting and disheartening information, what is one to do who wishes to lose body fat?

At the risk of sounding too simplistic, the only certitude we can draw from humans and energy (food) is that if you don't eat enough of it you will grow thinner and die (witness the phenomena of anorexia and the effects of food depravation on prisoners of war in World War II concentration camps), and if you eat lots and lots of it you will grow quite bounteous, your health will suffer, and you will also die. Knowing the realities of these two extremes, it would make sense to take stock of where you are now, which is probably somewhere in the middle of this spectrum, and, if your desire is to lose body fat, scale back your energy input a little bit (or quite a bit) from this point.

Whatever you are eating now—whether it's carbohydrate-rich foods, fatty foods, or high-protein foods—if you are carrying too much body fat, the sad reality is that you are probably eating too much. Your organs and cells all have specific nutrient needs, and your body fat likewise has needs for its survival. If you consider yourself to be storing too much fat you are simply inputting energy into your system at a rate over and above the needs of your organs and cells, thus allowing for the preservation (or expansion) of the fat colonies throughout your body. Scale your energy input back a bit for a little while and you will lose fat; scale it back a lot for a year or so and you'll completely transform your appearance.

There are some who would suggest to those who are carrying too much fat that it's not their doing (and thus not a shortcoming) that has resulted in their storing of unwanted body fat; that instead, such people have simply inherited a gene that made them fat, or they have "toxins" that have blocked their body's ability to process and eliminate fat, and that they simply need a "cleanse," or need to make their diet coordinate with their blood type, etc. Such people who suggest such psychologically pacifying nonsense are mistaken and are usually selling something. You don't need a cleanse or a detox (unless your liver has shut down); you simply need to *eat less*. No additional exercise is required over and above what I have indicated earlier in this book. How do I know this? Simply because I've conducted numerous fat-loss studies at my facility over the years, wherein no conventional "cardio" exercise was performed at all.

The first study we conducted involved 22 women and 11 men, with ages ranging from 25 to 64. The study lasted 10 weeks. No supplements or macronutrient emphasis/omission was involved, and the subjects instead were simply given a well-balanced but calorie-reduced diet composed of regular food that you can purchase from any supermarket. As far as exercise went, the subjects followed a once-a-week resistance-training program similar to the ones indicated in this book. Here are the results:

WEIGHT & FAT LOSSES

Total Weight Loss:	442.4 lbs
Greatest Weight Loss (Men):	43.2 lbs
Greatest Weight Loss (Women):	25.8 lbs
Average Weight Loss:	17.02 lbs
Total Pure Fat Loss:	405 lbs

Greatest Fat Loss (Men):	33.8 lbs
Greatest Fat Loss (Women):	23.6 lbs
Average Fat Loss (Men):	20.9 lbs
Average Fat Loss (Women):	13.2 lbs
Average Pure Fat Loss:	15.58 lbs

STRENGTH INCREASES (AFTER 10 WORKOUTS)

Lower Body (Men):	43.05%
Lower Body (Women):	43.73%
Upper Body (Men):	30.42%
Upper Body (Women):	32.51%
Average Overall Strength Increase:	35.46%
Average Lean Gain % (Men):	+6.21%
Average Lean Gain % (Women):	+4.52%
Total Lean Muscle Increase:	+132.8%
Overall Average Lean Muscle Gain:	+5.11%

Given that all of the subjects on this study had been training with me for over a year and, thus, were not beginners by any means, this level of lean (and strength) gain is considerable. Moreover, to my knowledge, never before in the history of fat loss and exercise has there ever been this much fat lost with so little exercise having been performed. In fact, when the results were compared to those from another group we studied that trained with more exercises, it was discovered that those who trained with the least amount of exercise lost more fat and gained more muscle than the higher volume of exercise group by a ratio of 2 to 1.

In terms of diet, the subjects on the studies consumed regular food—three meals a day, plus two snacks. And, in case you were wondering, we have successfully repeated the results of this study with several hundred more clients over the years, indicating that the requirements for losing fat are, for the most part, far more dependent upon one reducing one's calorie input than on increasing one's physical activity levels.

HEALTH BENEFITS

While this may be interesting from a fat loss perspective, what I found even more intriguing were the health benefits that followed employing a resistance-training program coupled with a calorie-reduced diet. Blood pressure medications were found to be no longer necessary (a sure sign of cardiovascular improvement) for 30 percent of the subjects who took part in the study; cholesterol medications were also found to be no longer necessary for the same 30 percent, and individuals who had been diagnosed with type I diabetes were found to require 70 percent less nightly insulin. Individuals who had come off of knee replacement surgery now found that they could literally bound up flights of stairs that otherwise had represented an insurmountable obstacle. Rather impressive results from a workout that lasted a fraction of the time than most individuals seeking to lose fat typically follow!

THE ROLE OF STRENGTH TRAINING IN FAT LOSS

Resistance training helped our subjects enormously in their quest to lose fat—not from the calories burned during their exercise sessions, which were modest at best, but in the calories burned afterward. Consider the following medical facts:

- Muscle is metabolically expensive tissue. It requires more calories at rest than any other tissue and is responsible for 70 percent of the calories burned on a daily basis. The more you have of it, the higher your BMR (fat-burning ability) will be.
- Muscle is the first casualty on most diets and on most exercise programs. If you do not engage in resistance-training exercise, you will lose muscle when you cut back on your food intake. If you use resistance exercise, but it is performed for too many exercises or too often, you will—again—lose muscle tissue.

Training harder but less frequently delivers a strong signal to your body that it requires all the muscle it can and resting sufficiently between workouts allows your body the time it requires to build such muscle. Indeed, as we've seen earlier, training too frequently can prevent your body from producing or even maintaining muscle tissue.

While exercise scientists have known the above facts for over 50 years, for some reason this information seldom filters out to those people with fat-loss aspirations. The dramatic success of our fat-loss program has resulted in it being added as a permanent part of our strength and fitness center's (Nautilus North, in Bracebridge, Ontario) curriculum for those who wish to lose body fat in a rational and time-efficient manner.

Outside of my own research in this regard, a study that was presented at the 17th European Congress on Obesity revealed the relative contributions of overeating and physical activity to the obesity epidemic in America.[2] The researchers tested 963 children and 1,399 adults in order to determine how many calories their bodies actually utilized during their day-to-day activities. After collecting this data, the researchers then determined how many calories would need to be consumed in order for both groups to maintain a stable bodyweight (the calculations were adjusted for children in order to take into account their normal level of growth and development). The researchers then examined data from a nationally representative survey (NHANES) that had recorded the weight of Americans during the 1970s and early 2000s in order to determine the actual weight gain of Americans over this period of time. Lastly, the researchers examined the national food supply data to determine the quantity of food consumed by Americans from the 1970s to the early 2000s. The data thus collected allowed the researchers to determine the calorie intake relative to the calories burned, allowing them to predict the rate of weight gain during this 30-year period. The results revealed that the predicted and actual increase in weight gain among children of nearly nine pounds matched exactly, which indicated that overconsumption was most likely responsible for any additional weight gain they might have displayed. The adults came in a little bit below the predicted number for weight gain—they gained 20 pounds over this same period of time rather than the predicted 23.8 pounds. The lead researcher of the study, Boyd Swinburn, who is the chair of population health and director of the World Health Organization Collaborating Centre for Obesity Prevention at Deakin University in Australia, concluded that, "This study demonstrates that the weight gain in the American population seems to be virtually all explained by eating more calories. It appears that changes in physical activity played a minimal role."[3]

You will recall that one of the primal impulses we have inherited from our hunter-gatherer ancestors is that if you happen upon some form of energy, consume it because it might not be there tomorrow. Such an attitude in an environment in which energy is scarce might well be the difference between life and death. However, that same attitude applied within our present-day environment where lots of energy is readily available results in overconsumption, and often leads to health problems such as obesity, high blood pressure, and type II (and type I) diabetes, which has put many of us on a fast track to a miserable (from the standpoint of health) existence. All of us are programmed to input energy whenever we can and we're going to have to rewire our programming through hyperconscious attention to energy input values if we're going to even have a chance at reducing our body fat levels.

While there are those who claim that "calories don't count," their reasoning has always struck me as spurious. Such people use the word "calorie" as if it were something intrinsic to the food itself, but food doesn't actually contain calories, it contains energy, and it is this energy that is quantified by a measurement called a "calorie." It was originally defined in physics as the quantity of energy required to raise the temperature of a kilogram of water by one degree centigrade. But all things contain energy, which is why if you place a pound of muscle in a device called a bomb calorimeter, it will give off 600 calories of energy, while a pound of fat will give off 3,500 calories of energy. Similarly, the foods we eat contain various amounts of energy (the amount of energy that they supply can, as we've seen above, be affected by certain genetic elements). A calorie, then, is simply a measurement of a quantity of energy. To therefore say that, "calories don't count" is nonsensical, as that is precisely and only what they do—they quite literally "count" a given quantity of energy. To hold such a view is tantamount to saying that measurement doesn't measure, or that degrees "don't count" on a thermometer or that inches and centimeters don't provide a precise gauge of dimension and distance to someone building a house. Try framing a house without measuring and see how well that goes for you. Similarly, calories do count as a measurement of energy consumption as, without knowing how much energy you are inputting into your system, it is impossible to know whether you're consuming too much or too little—in other words, whether your diet is moving you nearer to or further away from your goal of losing body fat. And while certain types of foodstuffs may release calories quicker or slower from the food in which they are contained (the popular 3,500 calories of Jellybeans vs. 3,500 calories of broccoli), the reality is that one can only come to know such a differential through the measurement of calories.

UNDERSTANDING THE FAT-LOSS PROCESS

As indicated, our bodies require energy to operate, and this energy is found within the various foods we eat. What we put into our mouths is synthesized in a variety of complex chemical processes and is then converted to energy in the form of Adenosine Triphosphate (ATP) and glucose to fuel basic biological work within the body. This basic work—all of the involuntary activity that keeps the machinery going, from our heart beating to our lungs breathing—is called our basal metabolism. The speed at which this process operates for each individual is called the basal metabolic rate (or BMR).

The BMR is the basic level of the body's daily energy (calorie) needs—and these needs are substantial. Indeed, we may input a couple of tons of food into our body over the course of a year but only gain (or lose) a single pound. And, to compound things, each individual's BMR, or rate of energizing, will be different owing to differences in height, weight (muscle to fat ratios), gender, respiration, sleep patterns, etc. But the BMR is only part of the story. Our daily activities—from picking up a coffee cup to working out—also require energy. One's total energy or calorie needs, then, are based upon his or her own personal BMR plus daily energy needs for voluntary activity. It is essential to know this total if one is to have any chance of having any control over one's body fat levels. There are formulas that have been offered in the past that claim to be able to accurately predict the calorie requirements for a person's BMR and activity levels, but these are more guesstimates than precise science. The problem with such approaches is that if the math is off even by a mere 14.5 calories a day (which is the equivalent of one potato chip), over a period of, say, 20 years that could result in you gaining an extra 30 pounds of fat. Nevertheless, there does exist a simple and reasonably accurate way to determine your specific BMR and your total daily maintenance level of calories. Mike Mentzer taught it to me, and it is very simple and accurate. Every day for five days write down every single thing you eat, from the amount of cream you put into your morning coffee to the quantity of dressing you put on your salad. It is important for accuracy that this five-day period be typical of your normal eating habits, so during this period don't scale back on the food that you would normally input into your body, as this will only result in a false average. In other words, don't change your diet during this five-day period. Your goal with this bit of recordkeeping is to find out what your daily average caloric intake is over a representative five-day period. Then, after each day is over, sit down with a calorie-counting book, calculate your total number of calories consumed for that day, and do this for five days. At the end of your five-day period, take these five sums, add them together, and divide that number by five. The resulting integer will be your daily average calorie intake. For example, let's say on Monday you consumed 2,500 calories. On Tuesday that number went up to 2,700. By Wednesday, it's the middle of the week, and you're getting tired and frustrated from your job. A friend takes you out for lunch and you find yourself eating more in the evening than you usually do. When you total up that day's calorie intake you are shocked to learn that you consumed 4,500 calories that day. On Thursday you are feeling a little guilty about your dietary aberration from the day before, and so you only consume 1,500 calories. By Friday you're back to normal, and you consume a more modest 2,500 calories.

In the above example, the five daily sums added together equal 13,700. When 13,700 is divided by five, the number the person in the above example comes away with is 2,740. This represents your *daily average caloric intake*. If over this five-day period you didn't gain or lose weight then this daily average caloric intake also represents your daily *maintenance need of calories*; i.e., the number of calories this individual requires to maintain your present bodyweight (not to lose weight, nor to gain weight, but to maintain his present weight). Therefore, this is a very important number to know, as it takes into account an individual's BMR and the amount of calories you typically burn as a result of your daily voluntary physical activity. It further takes into account such factors as whether or not the person is male or female, has more muscle or less muscle, or has a fast or a slow metabolism. Consequently, each daily maintenance estimate of calories will be unique for each person who calculates it and has no application to anyone other than that person.

Once you have determined your individual specific number of calories that you need to consume on a daily basis in order to maintain your weight, then, if you want to lose body fat, you must simply eat less than this number of calories on a daily basis. That is to say, that you must reduce this number of calories to a lower figure. There's no need to be drastic at the start; one can begin one's journey to fat loss simply by reducing one's daily calorie intake by a mere 500 calories.

Using the numebrs in the example above, let's assume that you wish to lose body fat. Your daily maintenance need of calories has been determined to be 2,740. So you scale back your caloric input by 500 calories to 2,240. Your body understands, however, that you require 2,740 to maintain its present mass and so in an effort to redress this imbalance it will now turn to its stored energy (body fat) to make up the difference between what is required to maintain your weight and the amount that you are now consuming. After seven days on this lower calorie intake, your body will have used up 3,500 calories from stored body fat for fuel (500 a day x seven days), which is generally considered to be the number of calories in one pound of fat. After one month on this rather modest calorie reduction, this person will have lost four pounds of fat (4 x 3,500). After a month, this number can be reduced further if so desired and the fat loss will continue.

It is important for health, as well as fat loss, that the diet one follows—whether one is dieting for fat loss or not—is balanced. A balanced diet, according to most reputable nutritional scientists, is composed of carbohydrates, protein, and fats, which can be found in meats, fruits and vegetables, dairy products, and grains and cereals.

A BALANCED DIET

It may be simplistic to say that a well-balanced diet is "a little bit of every-thing," but in fact, that's exactly what it is. Nutritionists have divided foods into six groups based upon their similarities in nutritive value and their role in the diet. A balanced diet, then, includes multiple servings from each of these various food groups each day. Here's how they break down:

1. Meat, poultry, dry beans, and nuts group: Two to three servings (this group would include fish and eggs as well). Note: A serving size is modest; i.e., in the case of meat, three ounces will suffice and would not include gravies or sauces.
2. Vegetables: Three to five servings.
3. Fruits: Two to four servings.
4. Milk, yogurt, and cheese group: Two to three servings of milk or two to three servings of cheese, butter, or ice cream.
5. Breads and cereals: Four or more servings.
6. Fats, oils, and sweets: Use sparingly.

There is also a "seventh category"—snacks—but it's inconsequential and unnecessary if you're well looked after in the first six groups, and is highly undesirable if your goal is to lose body fat. These six groups are not the be-all and end-all of eating and nutrition, but they do represent a very reliable guide to balanced food consumption. They are analyzed in much greater detail in books devoted to nutrition (not diet books) and individual adjustments can then be made to suit your basic needs, your additional needs for energy consumption (such as exercise or dur-ing pregnancy), foods that are available in your part of the country, and your lifestyle.

MACRONUTRIENTS

There are four macronutrients—carbohydrates, fats, proteins, and water. They are the body's only important sources of energy and they are there-fore used in great quantities. The carbohydrates, much maligned by cer-tain diet advocates, are actually the body's preferred source of fuel. They're stored in the muscles and liver in the form of energy-giving glycogen. Fat, stored in the muscles, under the skin, and around body organs, is the second-best source of energy. Protein, though it enjoys the most public-ity, is a poor energy provider at any time, and the body has no way of storing it. Water may be the most important of all of the macronutrients, as we can live for some time without protein, fat, and carbohydrate, but we can only last a few days without water.

CARBOHYDRATES

Carbohydrates are chemical compounds of sugar, starches, and cellu-lose (fiber) containing the elements of carbon, hydrogen, and oxygen. All foodstuffs are ultimately converted into glucose (blood sugar) by the time they are digested and hit the bloodstream, and glucose is the body's primary energy source. The molecules in food that are converted to glu-cose are called monosaccharides (individual molecules), disaccharides (pairs), and polysaccharides (three or more). The body can only absorb monosaccharides, and so it chemically breaks down di- and polysac-charides into the usable form. Glucose, fructose, and galactose are the only monosaccharides that find their way to the liver, where fructose and galactose are converted to glucose and used for energy. Sugar, because it contains readily usable glucose, is absorbed into the blood-stream very quickly. Starches need to be broken down and absorbed at a slower rate. Interestingly, the original source of the glucose doesn't matter in the slightest—glucose is glucose whether it comes from an ice cream soda or mashed potatoes. As a source of energy, however, pure sugar or honey are poor choices, as they are absorbed immediately and may give a "rush" of energy, but there is no enduring effect. The more complex carbohydrates found in starchy foods such as potatoes and peas take longer for the body to process and provide a more enduring energy source.

Ordinarily, there is less than a quarter of an ounce of glucose avail-able in the bloodstream at any one time. But the body has 10–12 ounces more in storage in the heart and muscle tissue. This reserve glucose is used during prolonged exercise.

FATS

Fats, or lipids, are chemical compounds that don't dissolve in water. Most fats (about 98 percent) are called triglycerides, of which some are saturated and come from animals, and some are unsaturated and come from plants. Fats are very caloric—about nine calories per gram. This is more than twice the calorie value of carbohydrates. Low-fat diets are very effective for trimming the pounds, but much of the fat consumed daily is hidden (in meat, milk, cheese, and nuts) and difficult to eliminate without excluding other valuable nutrients as well.

PROTEIN

Protein is organic material that, next to water, is the primary structural material of the body's cells and tissues. There are about 20 amino acids in protein and at least nine of these (the so-called "essential" amino acids) have to come from one's daily diet. But just as the body doesn't care where it gets its glucose, it isn't concerned about the source of its protein. In other words, beans are as good as meat. Nutritionist Ronald Deutsch once wrote that, "protein has become the dietary lure to which the consumer consistently rises, like a hungry trout on a quiet morning." There is truth in what he says. It's a fact, of course, that protein is absolutely essential for the growth and repair of the body's tissues, but it has yet to be proven that more than enough of any essential element of nutrition is better than merely enough.

According to the Mayo Clinic's Kristi Wempen, the minimum amount of daily protein intake to prevent deficiency for the average sedentary adult would be 0.8 grams per 2.2 pounds of bodyweight. So a person weighing 165 pounds would require 60 grams of protein per day. If you are in your forties or fifties and have not started strength training to correct this condition, then that number should be increased to 1 gram per 2.2 pounds of bodyweight. If you are active and building muscle, your daily protein intake should fall somewhere between 1.1 and 1.7 grams of protein for every 2.2 pounds of bodyweight.[4]

Yet I know young men who play hockey and/or work out with weights who eat 500 grams of protein a day thinking it will help them gain additional muscle and strength. The protein they're eating obviously contains calories just as fats and carbohydrates do, which is an important consideration in a fat-loss program as the excess is stored as fat, even when that extra protein comes from a high-quality source, such as steak. You would need to eat a little more than five pounds of steak to get 500 grams of protein, so if such a high protein intake were an absolute requirement for human health then one would have to eat a tremendous amount of food in order to meet it. Unfortunately, this amount of meat would also contain more than 8,000 calories and about 675 grams of fat.

WATER

Water is obviously important when you consider that the body is 60 percent water. Water not only contains valuable minerals but also it acts as a lubricant, a shock absorber between cells, a digestion aid, and also serves as the body's principle means of cooling itself, performing the essential job of maintaining a steady core temperature.

In the course of an average day the body loses water steadily, though much of this loss (about 50 percent) is unseen. On a hot day it's not uncommon to lose five to eight quarts of fluid, which, of course, must be replaced either by drinking liquids (again, it doesn't matter what you drink—with the exception of alcohol—nor does the temperature of the drink matter) or through water that is contained in the foods we would normally consume. A surprising amount of seemingly solid food contains a high percentage of water. Meats can be as much as half water while most fruits and vegetables are at least 70 percent water.

MICRONUTRIENTS

VITAMINS

Vitamins are organic substances that play a major role in the control of the body's metabolic processes. They help to process the macronutrients—carbohydrates, fats, and protein—and serve as aids to the body's self-produced enzymes (forming co-enzymes), which function as biochemical catalysts. The body cannot manufacture its own vitamins so these must be obtained from one's diet. And this is not difficult to achieve if you're eating a balanced diet because the daily vitamin requirement is one-eighth of a teaspoon. Interestingly, though nutritionists agree that vitamins are essential to good health, there is little agreement on which vitamins (if any) are the most important, what is the proper dosage, or who needs them. It does seem clear, however, that vitamins in any amount do *not* cure disease or provide *extra* health protection. I grant that it is possible that vegetarians or people on low-calorie diets may not get the Recommended Daily Allowance of certain vitamins. But even this is unlikely because the fat-soluble vitamins—A, D, E, and K—are stored in the body's fat and don't need to be consumed daily. The water-soluble vitamins—C and eight B vitamins—should be consumed daily, but they are very easy to acquire even in a moderately well-balanced diet. One other point, vitamins do *not* provide energy and there is absolutely no need to increase your vitamin intake even during heavy exercise.

MINERALS

Minerals are chemicals found in the soil that are passed on to humans through plants and animals. They are vital to our various life processes but are only required in small quantities. Their function is to activate hormones and prevent anemia, and they play a vital role in controlling the beating of our hearts and the contractions of our muscles. The minerals that we require the most of are sodium, magnesium, calcium, and potassium. Other minerals, such as iron, cobalt, and iodine, are needed in trace amounts. Most minerals can be obtained from the daily diet if that diet includes vegetables, fruits, grains, and dairy products.

REALISTIC EXPECTATIONS

It's important for motivational and educational purposes for people to understand that fat loss is not a rapid process. Most people will not lose more than a few ounces of fat a day even while on a very reduced-calorie diet. I've had clients come into my facility who sincerely were looking to lose 30 pounds of fat in five weeks—more than eight ounces a day! The impossibility of this can easily be illustrated. First, you must consider that each gram of stored body fat contains nine calories of energy and, secondly, that one ounce is the equivalent of 28 grams. One ounce of fat, therefore, possesses 252 calories (or 28 x 9). In order to lose eight ounces of fat in one day, one would have to burn up 2,016 calories. That means your daily food intake must be 2,016 calories lower than the number required to maintain your existing bodyweight. Now, a person who weighs 200 pounds and is moderately active might require on the order of 3,200 calories a day to maintain his weight (approximately 1,700 calories to fuel his BMR and perhaps another 1,500 to fuel voluntary activity).

Were such an individual to reduce his caloric intake to a mere 1,200 per day, he would obviously incur a deficit of 2,000 calories a day. But when the body uses fuel for activity, it is never just in the form of fat. Only the cardiac muscle, the heart, lives off of fat for energy. The body's voluntary muscles use sugar, fat, and sometimes even muscle or protein for energy, depending upon the nature of the activity and the state of the body. Most skeletal muscle activity, including resistance training, demands glycogen or stored sugar. If your caloric intake is too low or you are on a low-carbohydrate diet, your body will actually convert existing protein and/or muscle tissue into sugar for sustained high-intensity activity. Fat does not contain alanine (an amino acid found in muscle tissue) and, therefore, cannot be used for fueling demanding muscular work. Consequently, in such cases, the body will take alanine out of the muscles and transport it to the liver, where it will be converted to the glucose your body needs. This means that you risk the possibility of using up your own muscle (and thus reducing your BMR) if you cut your calories back too much.

If you have been reducing your calories over several months and still find that there is some body fat that you would like to rid yourself of, you might then be best advised to burn some additional calories through some supplemental physical activity rather than reducing your calorie intake further. However, now that we've seen how some activities can do you more harm than good, it would be best to choose your supplemental activity wisely. A caloric reduction of 500 calories per day plus an energy expenditure of approximately 250 calories a week, plus the additional muscle you will be building through your resistance training workouts could see you with a total deficit of 3,750 calories a week and result in the loss of slightly more than two additional pounds of fat in two weeks. That doesn't sound like much, but viewed over six months, that's a loss of over 12 pounds of pure body fat, which could transform the way you look.

It sounds easy—and it is easy—if you can discipline yourself and stay with it. At best, the ability of human beings to regulate their food intake is very poor (recall that we are almost programmed genetically to always be looking to input energy into our systems) and sedentary people almost always eat more than they need. Exercise can be important in weight control—that is, the right type of exercise—as it tends to decrease appetite, and the rise in body temperature that occurs during exercise also inhibits hunger. Physiologists and nutritionists agree that the intensity of the exercise is also important in calorie cost, and only muscular work, in whatever form, uses the body's energy. Sitting and thinking about exercise won't do a thing but help broaden your behind.

DIETS AND WHY THEY WORK

If the prospect of losing four to eight pounds a month doesn't sound that exciting, just remember that it took you a lot longer than this to gain the fat that you're now looking to lose. Fat goes on gradually and comes off gradually. It is the desire to lose a lot of fat quickly that causes most people to look to radical diets, as these types of diets usually suggest that if you follow them you will lose much more fat than what I've indicated. People, being people after all, want to lose all of their unwanted fat right away—rather than letting nature take its natural and much slower course. You must remember, however, that most diets work in the short run because, whatever they may promise about eating all you want, their main trick is to get you to *eat less*.

Psychologically, such diets quickly become boring and you tend to eat even less than the diet's suggested allowance. What the Paleo and most other diets do is reduce the carbohydrate intake to below 60 grams a day—and this does cause a substantial weight loss immediately. The reason why is that carbohydrates are the body's main source of energy. The low-carbohydrate diet forces the body to reach into itself for substitute forms of fuel—some of its protein and stored fat. This shift in internal chemical processes results in more waste products. These wastes activate the kidneys and they, in turn, respond by getting rid of the waste. This reduces the body's water content. This loss can conceivably add up to 10 pounds in a week—but it's almost all fluid. Since fat contains very little water, you won't be losing fat.

To give you some idea of how much energy stored body fat represents, consider the "typical" young American woman, at five feet, five inches, and 128 pounds. A little over 25 of her 128 pounds will be fat tissue. And this much fat has enough energy to meet all of her needs for roughly 45 days—even if she were to take in no food at all. It obviously takes a severe and prolonged energy shortage to make any progress in shedding a meaningful amount of excess fat.

WHAT IS OVERWEIGHT?

The body has a sophisticated system of storing fuel for later use—keeping the tank filled, in other words. That extra fuel, over and above the combined BMR/Energy Expenditure rate, is converted to fat (the few pounds mentioned above). The body is designed to store a certain amount of fat as an energy reserve (fat is an extremely compact fuel supply, providing more than twice as many calories per gram as either proteins or carbohydrates do), for insulation, for padding, and for the lean times. But these days, in the United States at least, there are relatively few lean times, so most of us simply end up storing this surplus energy as fat. This excess serves no useful purpose, it's potentially harmful, and it's certainly unsightly. It's what makes us overweight.

There are a number of different tables that give recommended weight ranges adjusted to height. These charts aren't of much value except to show the wide range of human variation. They do not take into consideration individual differences such as body composition, skeletal size, and body type (ectomorph, mesomorph, or endomorph), all of which have an influence on weight. These charts give arbitrary numbers and should be used only with that fact in mind, but, with or without a chart, you can tell if you're overweight. Subjectively, you know if you feel overweight and you can confirm your worst fears by looking at yourself in the mirror. Objectively, you can tell if your clothes are getting too tight and you can't see the scale. If you fall outside the upper ranges of any of the height-weight charts, you are overweight.

If you are 20 percent above the recommended weight on the charts, you are probably not just overweight, but obese—a dreaded word in our society. No matter how little your food intake exceeds your energy output, you're going to put on weight. When this imbalance goes on for a time, you get overweight; if it continues, you get badly overweight; and finally, if you don't put a stop to it, you will become obese. No matter the cause, if you are heavier than your "ideal" weight (usually your weight at age 20), you are overweight. If you are 20 percent above that weight you are obese, unless you're very muscular; and if you're 25 percent over, you are subjecting yourself to potential health problems, not the least of which is heart disease. If you can't remember your weight at 20 (or if you were overweight then), and you can't honestly tell by looking in the mirror, then the "pinch test" is a good measure of fatness. The fat deposits under the skin (basically) reflect the total fat stored throughout the body. One of the best places to pinch is the back of the arm right behind the triceps. It's a little hard to take this measurement by yourself, so you may want to ask a friend to help. With your arm hanging straight down, take hold of the skin with your thumb and forefinger at the midpoint between the elbow and the shoulder. Pull the pinched area away from the muscle. The fat will pull away with the skin. If you're a man under 30 the layer of fat and skin pinched away should measure less than six-tenths of an inch; for a woman, less than 1.1 inches. If you're a man over 30, the fold should be less than nine-tenths of an inch and for a woman, less than 1.25 inches. If the measurement is greater than it should be, you can consider yourself overweight. But don't let this scare you. It's something you *need* to know.

The desire to lose body fat is nationwide; however, the fact remains that the majority of individuals seeking to lose fat fail in their task simply by not understanding the mechanism by which fat is lost, opting instead to try fad diets or partake in the consumption of special herbs, minerals, and other supposedly "fat-burning" supplements, or to perform aerobic exercise for several sessions a week. These people are often disappointed that, after a promising start, their fat-loss goal seems further and further from reach. Ultimately, most of these individuals will fall off the wagon, giving up both the diet and the aerobics, and will end up fatter than they were before starting the regimen.

The reasons why such approaches typically end in failure are many, but two reasons stand out above all others. First, there is a difference between weight loss and fat loss, and anytime you cut back on macro-nutrients that your body needs (such as carbohydrates, fats, or proteins) then your diet will suffer an imbalance, and nature abhors imbalances. The body cannot survive without all of the nutrients that its survival requires. Consequently, you can only endure a diet in which a macro-nutrient is omitted for so long before the body rebels and you end up consuming more of the macronutrient than you did before.

Second, the reason that aerobic activities, per se, fail to strip much fat off the body is that one pound of fat can provide the body with sufficient fuel for up to 10 hours of continuous aerobic activity, with the result that four to five sessions per week on a treadmill, in aerobics class, or on a stepping machine will make use of little more than an ounce or two of fat tissue for fuel. You can perform aerobics until you are quite literally blue in the face, and still not lose much in the way of body fat.

In truth, the reason why our metabolisms slow down with each passing decade of age is because we lose an estimated 6.6 pounds of muscle every decade once we exit our twenties, and with those 6.6 pounds of muscle, so, too, go the number of calories per day they were causing our bodies to burn. However, if that muscle is put back on the body through resistance training, then our metabolism correspondingly increases.

EPILOGUE

I have attempted in the pages of this book to provide the reader with a validation for a minimalist approach to exercise. Does this mean that the world will stop revolving if you opt to train more frequently or that you should give up activities that you love, such as yoga or jogging? No. If such methods of exercise are the only thing between your using your muscles in a meaningful way and not doing anything, then by all means continue on with them. What I hope to have conveyed to the reader, particularly the reader who has no desire to spend the bulk of his or her life in the gym, is that there is a viable alternative to this that produces results. As I hope will be evident to the reader, one no longer needs to spend hours in the gym or on the roads to become fit and healthy, and I have provided a means by which this can be accomplished that should take a minimal amount of time out of one's weekly schedule, leaving the reader with more time to spend on the more important things in his or her life.

It is important to recognize that no one exercise or diet program is magical; some exercise programs will allow you to output high levels of energy for a time, but all eventually must yield to the C.E.P. No exercise program will make you super-healthy or super-fit; no nutritional supplement will bestow upon you immortality nor get you back onto Main Street from a diet that has driven you too far off the course of health. It is time for our fitness IQ to mature; it's time to put away childish beliefs and wishes and replace them with specific and appropriate knowledge regarding the role and value of exercise in our lives.

We must remember that with proper exercise we are engaging an organic—not a mechanical—process, which is not unlike growing a plant. We have our genetic endowment and potential (analogous to the bulb); we have our environment: sleep, nutrition, stress, etc. (analogous to the soil); and we have the requisite stimulus for growth—the workout (analogous to watering the plant). While each of these things is important in bringing about the desired result (the ultimate growth and health of the plant), by focusing too narrowly on any one aspect we tend to lose perspective of the bigger picture of the process. I know of personal trainers that wax euphoric about the process of how they exercise, which seems to me to be akin to focusing on the "process" of how one pours water out of the water pot and onto the plant (e.g., "it should be done slow, with a calm mind, steady breathing, etc."). I just don't know if, in the bigger picture, it really makes *that* much difference. Similarly, many people in the fitness community believe that you simply can't have enough intensity of effort, which, again, to me seems akin to pouring way too much water on the plant for it to be able to process it optimally. Likewise, one wouldn't dump three pounds of soil on top of the plant and expect it to survive, nor should the aspiring exercise devotee dump into his or her system needless amounts of supplements nor consume way too much (nor too little) food and expect to make optimal progress. Again, it's an organic process.

We might well hit upon a perfect exercise stimulus and, if that stimulus aligns just right with our recovery interval, our nutrition, our sleep, our stress levels, and our hormone levels, it will activate our bodies into growth. Again, you can diligently apply your reason to creating the "perfect" protocol (and don't misunderstand me, I think this to be a good thing) and it will be the perfect protocol to use—but only for a while until the C.E.P. kicks in again; i.e., everything works—but not forever.

Conversely, if we discover further down the road that a given exercise program isn't prompting our bodies to produce any additional change, it may well be that our "plants" have already reached full bloom. This may also be a good thing, as it's not often that one knows in advance the consequences of an action. Perhaps there is a reason that nature decided that it should limit the amount of muscle mass that a normal human being can grow, or the aerobic capacity of the human organism. I've known many champion bodybuilders from the 1970s who now are either dead or very unhealthy (not all of them, by any means, but enough to give one pause).

Knowing that our bodies are economists with our energy systems, and that irrespective of what we do physically, they will, over time, figure out a way for us to accomplish what we are doing with less energy (muscular involvement), it might well explain the huge controversies over which is the "best way" to exercise for best results. Could it be that they are all the "best" ways for a limited amount of time?

We are often given the example of an athlete or celebrity who trains in a certain way and this is then held up as *the best* way to exercise, when in reality it might simply represent a hitching post on that particular individual's forthcoming encounter with the C.E.P. Still, being a member of the problem-solving species, it compels those of us who wish to exercise in an efficient, productive, and rational way to understand what science has found to be the underlying cause of the benefits we seek. In other words, if we're going to "water our plant," we want to make sure that the water we're applying isn't too much, too little, or contains chemicals or elements that will do our plant more harm than good.

The importance of exercise has been grossly overexaggerated for commercial purposes almost since its inception, resulting in more harm than good being done to countless souls who only wanted to be fitter. People have busy lives these days. They don't have time to waste in the gym that could be spent with their loved ones or on other ways of improving their station in what we've come to understand is an all-too-brief existence. If nothing else, hopefully the information I have provided the reader has allowed him or her to see that the proper way to view exercise is as an adjunct to his or her life, and not as the reason for it.

I began this book citing a dialogue I shared with my late friend Mike Mentzer, and so perhaps it is only fitting that I end it with a quote from him as well. I know that there will be those people who simply choose to ignore the facts and data that I have presented herein. To many, this information will represent something that threatens their worldview when it comes to keeping alive their dream that they can become something other than what their genetics will allow. And while Mike was speaking specifically about the desire to build larger muscles, the sentiment he expressed is applicable to the obsession many people have about anything, and their willingness to abandon reason and reality in their quest to follow the false gods that have been set before us by the exercise industry:

> He who acts contrary to what his perceptions and rational thoughts tell him is the truth is akin to Dostoevsky's Underground Man who cries: "What do I care for the laws of nature and arithmetic, when, for some reason, I don't like them, or the fact that two plus two equals four?" It's up to you.

NOTES ON TEXT

INTRODUCTION

1. U.S. Department of Health and Human Services, National Center for Health Statistics. 1977. National Health Examination Survey I: 1959–1962. Washington, D.C.: U.S. Department of Health and Human Services, National Center for Health Statistics, producer; Ann Arbor: Inter-University Consortium for Political and Social Research, distributor; U.S. Department of Health and Human Services, National Center for Health Statistics. Survey IIII. Washington, D.C.: U.S. Department of Health and Human Services, National Center for Health Statistics, producer; Ann Arbor: Inter-University Consortium for Political and Social Research, distributor; Centers for Disease Control. 2003. National Health and Nutrition Examination Survey. Available at http://www.cdc.gov/nchs/nhanes.htm.Health; Cutler, David M., Glaeser, Edward L., Shapiro, Jesse M., Why Have Americans Become More Obese? *Journal of Economic Perspectives* – Volume 17, Number 3, Summer 2003, pp. 93–118.

2. http://money.usnews.com/money/personal-finance/articles/2013/01/02/the-heavy-price-of-losing-weight

CHAPTER ONE

1. http://www.time.com/time/magazine/article/0,9171,1914974,00.html

2. Votruba, S.B., "The role of exercise in the treatment of obesity." *Nutrition* 16 (2000): 179–88.

3. Yale J.-F., et al., "Metabolic responses to intense exercise in lean and obese subjects." *J Clin Endocrin Metab* 68 (1989): 438–45.

4. Timmon, J.A., et al., "Using molecular classification to predict gains in maximal aerobic capacity following endurance exercise training in humans." *J Appl Physiol* 108 no.6 (Jun. 2010):1487–96. doi: 10.1152/japplphysiol.01295.2009. Epub 2010 Feb 4.

5. http://www.dailymail.co.uk/health/article-2255867/Is-minutes-week-exercise-need-fit-Scientists-say-ideal-fitness-regime-involves-intense-bursts-activity.html

6. In England: http://www.birmingham.ac.uk/news/latest/2011/08/01Aug-Less-than-ten-minutes-of-intense-exercise-a-week-is-enough-to-reduce-risk-of-cardiovascular-disease-and-diabetes-according-to-new-research.aspx; in Canada: http://well.blogs.nytimes.com/2012/02/15/how-1-minute-intervals-can-improve-our-health/

7. Morris, J.N., Heady, J.A., Raffle, P.A.B., Roberst, C.G., and Parks, J.W., "Coronary Heart Disease and Physical Activity of Work." *Lancet* 2 (1953): 1053–1057, 1111–1120.

8. Tzankoff S.P., Norris A.H., "Longitudinal changes in basal metabolic rate in man." *J. Appl. Physiol.*, 33 (1978), 538–539.

CHAPTER TWO

1. http://demog.berkeley.edu/-andrew/1918/figure2.html

2. Bridges P.S. "Degenerative joint disease in hunter-gatherers and agriculturists from the southeastern United States." *Am J Phys Anthropol.*, 1991 Aug; 85 (4): 379–91.

3. http://longevity.about.com/od/longevitystatsandnumbers/a/Longevity-Throughout-History.htm

4. http://www.cbc.ca/news/health/life-expectancy-in-canada-hits-80-for-men-84-for-women-1.2644355

5. Clement, D.B., Taunton, J.E., Smart, G.W., McNicol, K.L., "A survey of Overuse Running Injuries." *Physician and Sports Medicine* 9, no. 5 (May 1981): 547–558. A more recent survey of long-distance runners injuries puts the percentage of injuries on a scale that moves from 19.4 percent to 92.4 percent; van Gent, R.N., Siem, D., van Middlekoop, M., van Os, A.G., Bierma-Zeinstra, S.M.A., and Koes, B.W., Incidence and determinants of lower extremity running injuries in long distance runners: a systematic review, *Br J Sports Med*

2007 41:469–480 originally published online May 1, 2007 doi: 10.1136/bjsm.2006.033548

6. Solomon, Henry. *The Exercise Myth*, p. 99.

7. http://www.success.com/article/from-the-corner-office-dr-kenneth-cooper

8. Cooper, K.H., in *Prevention and Rehabilitation in Ischemic Heart Disease*. (Long, C., ed.) Baltimore: Williams & Wilkins, 1980.

9. Sullivan, D.J., "Stress Fractures In Runners." Paper presented at meeting of the American College of Surgeons, Chicago, Oct. 1982.

10. http://www.ama-assn.org/amednews/2012/06/18/hlsa0618.htm

11. O'Keefe, J.H., et al., "Potential adverse cardiovascular effects from excessive endurance exercise." *Mayo Clinic Proceedings* 87 no. 6 (Jun 2012) 587–95. doi: 10.1016/j.mayocp.2012.04.005.

12. Solomon, Henry A., "The Exercise Myth: Excessive Exercise Can Harm Your Health!" *EnCognitive*, http://encognitive.com/node/3972

13. Ibid.

14. Ibid.

CHAPTER THREE

1. Karavirta, L.; Hakkinen, K.; Kauhanen, A.; Arija-Blazquez, A.; Sillanpaa, E.; Rinkinen, N.; Hakkinen, A., "Individual responses to combined endurance and strength training in older adults." *Med Sci Sports Exerc.* 2011 Mar; 43 (3): 484–90. Doi:10.1249/MSS.0b013e3181f1bf0d.

2. Timmons, J.A., "Variability in training-induced skeletal muscle adaptation." *J Appl Physiol*, 110 no. 3 (Mar. 2011) 846–53. Doi; 10.1152/japplphysiol.00934.2010. Epub 2010 Oct 28.

3. "The Workout Enigma," November 17, 2010, online edition of the *New York Times:* https://well.blogs.nytimes.com/2010/11/17/phys-ed-the-workout-enigma/

CHAPTER FOUR

1. Hausenblas, Heather A., and Katherin Schrieber, "Addiction to Exercise," *BMJ*, April 26, 2017; 357; j1745.

2. Ibid.

3. http://www.oregonlive.com/ducks/index.ssf/2017/01/oregon_
    ducks_workouts_hospital.html

CHAPTER FIVE

1. www.runningroom.com/hm/inside.php?id=2669
2. Whyte, et al, "Ultra-endurance exercise and oxidative damage: impli-
    cations for cardiovascular health." *Med Sci Sports Ecerc*, 33 no. 5
    (May 2001) 850–851. "Echocardiographic studies report cardiac dys-
    function following ultra-endurance exercise in trained individuals.
    Ironman and half-Ironman competition resulted in reversible abnor-
    malities in resting left ventricular diastolic and systolic function.
    Results suggest that myocardial damage may be, in part, responsible
    for cardiac dysfunction, although the mechanisms responsible for
    this cardiac damage remain to be fully elucidated;" Knez, W.L. et al.
    Sports Med. 36(5): 429–41 (2006); Sherman J.E. et al., "Endurance
    exercise, plasma oxidation and cardiovascular risk." *Acta Cardiol.*
    Ded; 59 (6): 636–42 (2004); Shern-Brewer R, et al., "Exercise and
    cardiovascular disease: a new perspective." *Arterioscler Thomb Vasc
    Biol.* Jul; 18(7): 1181–7 (1998).
3. Swanson, D.R., "Atrial fibrillation in athletes: implicit literature-
    based connection suggest that overtraining and subsequent inflam-
    mation may be a contributing mechanism." *Med Hypotheses*: 2006;
    66(6): 1085–92.
4. Deichmann et al, *Melanoma Res.* June 2001; 11 (3): 291–6. "In meta-
    static melanoma S100beta [a marker of cancer] as well as melanoma
    inhibitory activity (MIA) are elevated in the serum in the majority of
    patients. Elevation has been found to correlate with shorter survival,
    and changes in these parameters in the serum during therapy were
    recently reported to predict therapeutic outcome in advanced dis-
    ease." Santos et al, *Life Sci.*, 17 no. 16 (Sep. 2004) 1917–1924, "After
    the test (a 30km run), athletes from the control group presented an
    increase in plasma CK (4.4-fold), LDH (43%), PGE2 6.6-fold) and
    TNF-alpha [another marker of cancer] (2.34-fold) concentrations,
    indicating a high level of cell injury and inflammation."
5. Wu, H.J., *World J Gastroenterol.*, 10 no. 18 (Sep. 2004) 2711–2714.

"RESULTS: Total bilirubin (BIL-T), direct bilirubin (BIL-D), alkaline phosphatase (ALP), aspartate aminotransferase (AST), alanine aminotransferase (ALT) and lactate dehydrogenase (LDH) increased statistically significantly ($P<0.05$) the race. Significant declines ($P<0.05$) in red blood cell (RBC), hemoglobin (Hb) and hematocrit (Hct) were detected two days and nine days after the race. 2 days after the race, total protein (TP), concentration of albumin and globulin decreased significantly. While BIL, BIL-D and ALP recovered to their original levels. High-density lipoprotein cholesterol (HDL-C) remained unchanged immediately after the race, but it was significantly decreased on the second and ninth days after the race. CONCLUSION: Ultra-marathon running is associated with a wide range of significant changes in hematological parameters, several of which are injury related. To provide appropriate health care and intervention, the man who receives athletes on high frequent training program high intensity training programs must monitor their liver and gallbladder function." [Note: HDL is lowered, LDL is increased. Red blood cell counts and white blood cell counts fall. The liver is damaged and gall bladder function is decreased. Testosterone decreases.]

6. Warhol et al., *Am J Pathol.* 118 no. 2 (Feb. 1985) 331–339. "Muscle from runners showed post-race ultrastructural changes of focal fiber injury and repair: intra and extracellular edema with endothelial injury; myofibrillar lysis, dilation and disruption of the T-tubule system, and focal mitochondrial degeneration without inflammatory infiltrate (1–3 days). The mitochondrial and myofibrillar damage showed progressive repair by 3–4 weeks. Late biopsies showed central nuclei and satellite cells characteristic of the regenerative response (8–12 weeks). Muscle from veteran runners showed intercellular collagen deposition suggestive of a fibrotic response to repetitive injury. Control tissue from non-runners showed none of these findings."

7. Neyiackas and Bauer, *South Med J.* 74 no. 12 (1981) 1457–60, "All post race urinalyses were grossly abnormal . . . We conclude that renal function abnormalities occur in marathon runners and that the severity of the abnormality is temperature-dependent."

8. Fagerhol et al. *Scan J Clin Invest*. 2005; 65 no. 3 (2005) 211–20 (2005), "During the marathon, half-marathon, the 30-km run, the ranger-training course and the VO2max exercise, calprotectin levels increased 96.3-fold, 13.3-fold, 20.1-fold, 7.5-fold and 3.4-fold, respectively. These changes may reflect damage to the tissues or vascular endothelium, causing microthrombi with subsequent activation of neutrophils."

9. Marchi et al., *Restor Neurol Neurosci*, 21 nos. 3–4 (2002) 109–21, "S100beta in serum is an early marker of BBB openings that may precede neuronal damage and may influence therapeutic strategies. Secondary, massive elevations in S100beta are indicators of prior brain damage and bear clinical significance as predictors of poor outcome or diagnostic means to differentiate extensive damage from minor, transient impairment." [Note: This damage resembles acute brain trauma, indicating elevated levels of S100beta, which is a marker of brain damage and blood brain barrier dysfunction.]

10. Schmitt et al., *Int J Sports Med*, 26 no. 6 (Jul. 2005) 457–63, "The aim of this study was to assess bone mineral density (BMD) and degenerative changes in the lumbar spine in male former elite athletes participating in different track and field disciplines and to determine the influence of body composition and degenerative changes on BMD. One hundred and fifty-nine former male elite athletes (40 throwers, 97 jumpers, 22 endurance athletes) were studied. . . . Throwers had a higher body mass index than jumpers and endurance athletes. Throwers and jumpers had higher BMD (T-LWS) than endurance athletes. Bivariate analysis revealed a negative correlation of BMD (T-score) with age and a positive correlation with BMD and Kellgren score ($p < 0.05$). Even after multiple adjustment for confounders lumbar spine BMD is significantly higher in throwers, pole vaulters, and long- and triple jumpers than in marathon athletes."

11. Srivastava, A., Kreiger, N., "Relation of physical activity to risk of testicular cancer." *Am J Epidemiol*. 151 (2000) 78–87.

12. Paffenbarger, R.S. Jr., Hyde, R.T., and Wing, A.L., "Physical activity and incidence of cancer in diverse populations: a preliminary report." *Am J Clin Nutr* 45 suppl. 1 (1987), 312–17.

13. Polednak, A.P., "College athletics, body size, and cancer mortality." *Cancer* 38 (1976) 382–387.

14. www.sciencedaily.com/releases/2015/06/150616093646.htm

15. Some samples of deaths reported to have occurred during a 10k run: http://m.scotsman.com/news/father-34-collapsed-and-died-minutes-from-10k-race-finishing-line-1-1544958; http://yourhealth.asiaone.com/content/25-year-old-woman-dies-after-running-10km-marathon; http://www.ncbi.nlm.nih.gov/m/pubmed/20086407/ http://m.independent.ie/irish-news/woman-24-died-of-heatstroke-in-10k-run-26136058.html. Some journals devoted to running point out that in many instances a preexisting heart condition may have been present (e.g., http://www.runnersworld.com/health/can-you-prevent-sudden-death?page=single and http://www.sportsscientists.com/2009/10/3-runners-die-in-detroit-safety-of/), but this simply makes my point for me—such activities as running a 10k do NOT provide special dispensation or protection from existent heart disorders and there is some evidence that running, particularly long distances, can actually damage the heart (http://www.dailymail.co.uk/health/article-2627279/How-craze-running-longer-distances-DAMAGE-heart.html; http://www.medicalnewstoday.com/articles/267305.php, http://www.mayoclinicproceedings.org/article/S0025-6196(12)00473-9/abstract).

16. *J Am Coll Cardiol.* 2014; 64(5):472–481. doi:10.1016/j.jacc.2014.04.058

17. Garber, C.E., Blissmer, B., Deschenes, M.R., et al., "Quantity and quality of exercise for developing and maintaining cardiorespiratory, musculoskeletal, and neuromotor fitness in apparently healthy adults: guidance for prescribing exercise," *Med Sci Sports Exerc.* 2011; 43 no. 7 (2010) 1334–59; Gibala, M.J., Little, J.P. "Just HIT it! A time-efficient exercise strategy to improve muscle insulin sensitivity." *J Physiol.*, 588 (18): 3341–2. (2010); Gibala, M.J., Little, J.P., Essen, M.V., et al. "Short-term sprint interval versus traditional endurance training: similar initial adaptations in human skeletal muscle and exercise performance." *J Physiol.* 575, no. 3 (2006) 901–11.; Haltom, R., Kraemer, R.R. Sloan, R.A., Frank, K., Tryniecki, J.L., "Circuit weight

training and its effects on excess postexercise oxygen consumption." *Med Sci Sports Exerc*, 31 (1999) 1202–7 (1999); Kravitz, L. "The fitness professional's complete guide to circuits and intervals." *IDEA Today*,14 no. 1 (1996) 32–43.; Murphy, E., Schwarzkopf, R. "Effects of standard set and circuit weight training on excess post-exercise oxygen consumption." *J Strength Cond Res*. 1992;6(2):66–124; Tabata, I., Nishimura, K., Kouzaki, M., *et al*. "Effects of moderate-intensity endurance and high-intensity intermittent training on anaerobic capacity and VO2max." *Med Sci Sports Exerc*, 28(10):1327–30. (1996); Trapp, E.G., Chisholm, D.J., Fruend, J., Bouthcher, S.H., "The effects of high-intensity intermittent exercise training on fat loss and fasting insulin levels of young women." *Int J Obes*., 32no. 4 (2008) 684–91.

18. http://www.jssm.org/vol11/n3/17/v11n3-17pdf.pdf
19. http://www.ncbi.nlm.nih.gov/pmc/articles/PMC2803113/
20. http://www.mayoclinic.or/healthy-lifestyle/fitness/expert-answers/heart-rate/faq-20057979
21. Burgomaster, K.A., Hughes, S.C., Heigenhauser, G.J.F., Bradwell, S.N., and Gibala, M.J. "Six sessions of sprint interval training increases muscle oxidative potential and cycle endurance capacity in humans." *J Appl Physiol*, 98: 1985–1990 (2005); Coyle, E.F.; "Very intense exercise-training is extremely potent and time efficient: a reminder." *J Appl Physiol*, 98 no. 6 (June 1, 2006) 1983–1984.
22. https://csus-dspace.calstate.edu/handle/10211.3/139453.
23. King, N., Hopkins, M., Caudwell, P., Stubbs, J., and Blundell, J. "Beneficial effects of exercise: shifting the focus from body weight to other markers of health." *The British Journal of Sports Medicine*, doi:10.1136/bjsm.2009.065557
24. http://well.blogs.nytimes.com/2009/11/04/phys-ed-why-doesn't-exercise-lead-to-weight-loss/
25. www.dailymail.co.uk/sciencetech/article-3276926/The-pointlessness-long-distance-runner.html

CHAPTER SIX

1. Chaya, M.S., Kurpad, A.V., Nagendra, H.R., et al., "The effect of

long term combined yoga practice on the basal metabolic rate of healthy adults," *BMC Complementary and Alternative Medicine*, vol. 6, no 28, published online August 21 2006 (www.biomedcentral. com/1472–6882/6/28.)

2. http://www.health.gov.au/internet/main/publishing.nsf/ content/0E9129B3574FCA53CA257BF0001ACD11/$File/ Natural%Therapies%20Overview%20Report%20Final%20with%20 copyright%2011%20March.pdf; pages 141–157.

3. Ibid., 156.

4. Embolism ("Fatal Air Embolism after Yoga Breathing Exercises," *Journal of the American Medical Association*, 210. No. 10 (Dec. 8, 1969), 1923.

5. Reinhold Ganz, an orthopedic surgeon at the University of Berne, in Switzerland claimed that between 2001 and 2008 his team published many studies, the one in 2008 indicating that women between 30 and 40 years of age whose activities made "high demands on motion" inclined toward hip damage more frequently. The paper specifically cited yoga as a contributing factor. (http://mobile.nytimes. com/2013/11/03/sunday-review/womens-flexibility-is-a-liability-in-yoga.html?_r=1&referer=http://yogalign.com/yoga-injuries-2/)

6. Ibid.

7. Ibid.

8. Sinaki, M., "Yoga Spinal Flexion Position and Vertebral Compression Fracture in Osteopenia or Osteoporosis of Spine: Case Seres." *Pain Practice.* (Mar. 26, 2012).

9. Matsushita, T. et al., *Biopsychosoc Med.*, 9, no. 9 (Mar. 18, 2015). doi:10.1186/s13030-015-0037-1.eCollection 2015.

10. *New York Times* article: http://www.nytimes.com/2012/01/08/maga-zine/how-yoga-can-wreck-your-body.html?_r=0.

11. http://www.cracked.com/article_19283_7-ancient-forms-mysti-cism-that-are-recent-inventions.html

12. SafeKidsUSA website: http://www.usa.safekids.org/tier3_cd.cfm? folder_id=540&content_item_id=12111

13. Thacker, Stephen B., et al., "The Impact of Stretching on Sports Injury RiskL a Systematic Review of the Literature." *Medicine and Science in Sports and Exercise*, 36 no. 3 (Mar. 2004): 371–8.

14. "New Study Links Stretching with Higher Injury Rates," *Running Research News*, Vol. 10(3), pp. 5–6, 1994.

15. Herbert, Rob D., and Gabriel, Michael., "Effects of Stretching Before and After Exercising on Muscle Soreness and Risk of Injury: Systematic Review." *BMJ*, 325:482 (2002).

16. Pope, R.P., et al., "A Randomized Trial of Pre-Exercise Stretching for Prevention of Lower Limb Injury," *Medicine & Science in Sports & Exercise*, 32:271 (2000).

17. http://saveyourself.ca/bibliography.php?her00

18. Witvrouw, E., et al. "The role of stretching in tendon injuries." *Br J Sports Med*. 41:226–226 (2007).

19. http://well.blogs.nytimes.com/2009/11/25/physed-how-necessary-is-stretching.

20. Ibid.

21. Nelson, Arnold G., et al., "A Single Thirty Second Stretch is Sufficient to Inhibit Maximal Voluntary Strength," *Medicine & Science in Sports & Exercise*, 38, no. 5 (May 2006), S294.

22. Peak Performance 46 (Jul 1994). Research carried out at the University of Hawaii, runners who stretched regularly were about 33 percent more likely to be injured compared to those who never stretched.

23. http://www.ncbi.nlm.nih.gov/m/pubmed/19918196/?i=/22266545/related.

CHAPTER SEVEN

1. Kelly, Friery, and Bishop, Phillip., "Long-Term Impact Of Athletic Participation On Physical Capabilities." *Journal of Exercise Physiologyonline (JEPonline)*. 10, no.1 (Feb. 2007).

2. Children's Hospital Boston web page: http://www.childrenshospital.org/az/Site1112/printerfriendlypageS1112P0.html

3. SafeKidsUSA website: http://www.usa.safekids.org/tier3_cd.cfm?folder_id=540&content_item_id=1211

4. Some of the studies reviewed in this research included: Brown, E.W., and Kimball, R.S., "Medical history associated with adolescent powerlifting." *Pediatrics 72*:636–644.1983; Kristiansen, B. "Association football injuries in schoolboys." *Scand. J. Sports Sci.* 5(1):1–2.1983; McCracken, P., "Will rugby scar your child for life?" *Personality*

Magazine (South Africa). pp. 18–20. May 1989; Ryan, J.R, and Salciccioli, G.G., "Fractures of the distal radial epiphyses in adolescent weightlifters." *Am. J. Sports;* Sparks, J.P., "Half a million hours of Rugby football." *Br. J. Sports Med.* 15:30–32.1981; Zaricznyj, B., et al., "Sports related injuries in school aged children." *Am. J. Sports.*

5. Hamill, B.P., "Relative safety of weightlifting and weight training." *J. Strength and CondoRes.* 8(1):53–57 (1994).

6. Schmidtbleicher, D., "An interview on strength training for children." *Nat. Strength Condo Assoc. Bulletin,* 9(12):42a-42b.1988.

CHAPTER EIGHT

1. Mursu, Jaako, et al., "Dietary Supplements and Mortality Rate in Older Women." *Arch Intern Med.* 2011;171(18):1625–1633. doi:10.1001/archinternmed.2011.445.

2. Klein, Eric A., et al., "Vitamin E and the Risk of Prostate Cancer (The Selenium and Vitamin E Cancer Prevention Trial (Select)." *JAMA.* 306, no.14 (2011) 1549–1556. doi:10.1001/jama.2011.1437

3. www.journals.plos.org/plosmedicine/article?id=10.1371/journal.pmed.0020168

4. www.nlm.hih.gov/medlineplus/druginfo/natural/1001.html

5. www.atbcstudy.cancer.gov

6. www.mayoclinic.org/drugs-supplements/vitamin-a/safety/hrb-20060201

7. www.https://ods.od.nih.gov/factsheets/VitaminB6-Consumer/

8. Cramer, J.K., et al., "Post-exercise Glycogen Recovery and Exercise Performance Is not Significantly Different Between Fast Food and Sport Supplements." *J Sport Nutr Exerc Metab.* 25, no. 5 (Mar. 26, 2015) 448–55. www.ncbi.nlm.nih.gov/m/pubmed/25811308/

9. Linde, C., Gadler, F., Kappenberger, L., and Rydén, L., "Placebo effect of pacemaker implantation in obstructive hypertrophic cardiomyopathy." *Am J Cardiol,* 83, no. 6 (Mar. 15, 1999) 903–907.

CHAPTER NINE

1. http://www.muscleandfitness.com/workouts/arms-exercises/build-arms-arnold-schwarzenegger

2. http://www.bodybuildingology.com/arnold-training.shtml

3. Rogers, R.A., et al., "The Effect of Supplemental Isolated Weight Training Exercises on Upper Arm Size and Upper Body Strength." *Journal of Strength & Conditioning Research*, 14, no. 3 (Aug. 2000), 369. The aim of this study was to examine the hypothesized additional training effect of programming isolated supplemental exercises in conjunction with compound weight-training exercises on muscle size and strength. Seventeen national-level baseball players volunteered to partite in this 10-week training study and were randomly divided into two groups. The control group completed a 10-week training program consisting of the bench press, lat pull-down, dumbbell incline press, and dumbbell 1-arm row exercises. The treatment group completed the same training program but with the addition of biceps curl and triceps extension exercises. A tape measure was used to record upper-arm circumferences, and a 5 repetition maximum (5RM) was determined on the bench press and lat pull-down for each subject before and after training. Both the treatment and control groups displayed significant increases in upper-arm circumference (6.6 and 6.5 percent, respectively), 5RM bench press (21.4 and 22.1 percent, respectively) and 5RM lat pull-down (15.7 and 14.5 percent, respectively). There were no significant differences between the groups in the percentage change before and after training. The findings of this study suggest that isolation exercises are not necessary in order to increase compound movement strength or increase upper-arm girth. These findings also suggest that strength coaches can save time by not including isolation exercises and still achieve increases in strength and size.

4. Lee, S.J., "Regulation of Muscle Mass by Myostatin." *Annu Rev Cell Dev Biol.* 20 (2004) 61–86.

5. Stewart, C.E.H., and Rittweger, J., "Adaptive processes in skeletal muscle: Molecular regulators and genetic influences." *J Musculoskelet Neuronal Interact* 2006; 6: 73–86.

6. Van Etten, L.M.L.A., Verstappen, F.T.J., and Westerterp, K.R., "Effect of body build on weight-training-induced adaptations in body composition and muscular strength." *Med Sci Sports Exerc* 26 (1994) 515–21.

7. www.ncbi.nlm.nih.gov/m/pubmed/26428621/

8. www.forbes.com/sites/alexmorrel/2015/03/12lawsuits-say-protein-powders-lack-protein-ripping-off-athletes/

9. www.nature.com/bjc/journal/v112/n7/full/bjc201526a.html

10. https://news.brown.edu/articles/2015/04/muscles

11. http://link.springer.com/article/10.1007/s00421-015-3243-4?wt_mc=alerts.TOCjournals

12. MacDougall, J.D., et al., "Biochemical adaptation of human skeletal muscle to heavy resistance training and immobilization." *J. Appl Phyisol.: Respirat. Enivorn. Exerc. Physiol.* 43(1977) 700–703; Tesh, P.A., Colliander, E.B., and Kaiser., P. "Muscle metabolism during intense, heavy-resistance exercise." *Eur. J. Appl. Physiol.* 55 (1986) 362–366; Piehl, K., "Glycogen storage and depletion in human skeletal muscle fibers." *Acta Physiol. Scand. (Suppl.)* 402 (1974) 1–32; Tesh, Per A., "Skeletal muscle adaptation consequent to long-term heavy resistance exercise," *Medicine and Science in Sports and Exercise.* 20, no. 5 (1988) S133.

CHAPTER TEN

1. Lombardo, Michael P., and Deaner, Robert O., "You Can't Teach Speed: Sprinters Falsify the Deliberate Practice Model of Expertise." *PeerJ* 2 (2014), 445. http://papers.ssrn.com/sol3/papers.cfm?abstract_id=2277977.

2. http://mobile.journals.lww.com/nsca-jscr/_layouts/oaks.journals.mobile/articleviewer.aspx?year=2011&issue=09000&article=00027

CHAPTER ELEVEN

1. www.latimes.com/science/sciencenow/la-sci-sn-laziness-imperative-exercise-calories-20150910-story.html

2. Ogasawara, Riki, et al., "mTOR Signaling Response to Resistance Exercise is Altered by Chronic Resistance Training and Detraining in Skeletal Muscle," *Applied Physiology* 114 no. 7 (2013), 934–40.

3. Pontzer, Herman, et al., "Constrained Total Energy Expenditure and Metabolic Adapation to Physical Activity in Adult Humans," *Current Biology*, 26, no. 3 (2016) 410–417, DOI: 10.1016/j.cub.2015.12.046

4. http://www.ncbi.nlm.nih.gov/pmc/articles/PMC2647711/
5. http://www.bloomberg.com/news/articles/2016-01-28/ more-exercise-doesn-t-always-mean-losing-weight

CHAPTER TWELVE

1. Warburton, Darren, Nicol, Crystal Whitney, and Bredin, Shanon., "Health Benefits of Physical Activity: The Evidence." *Canadian Medical Association Journal* 174 (2006): 801–9.

2. Researchers studied patients with advanced melanoma to understand the illness as it related to muscle strength. They looked at CT scans of the psoas muscle in order to measure core muscle density. The authors then correlated the core muscle density with the risk of metastasis, or spreading of the cancer. Patients with higher muscle density were found to have significantly better survival rates and less metastasis. The authors concluded that decreased muscle density was an important predictor in the outcome of the disease. Furthermore, they stated that "frailty, not age, was associated with decreased disease-free survival."

3. Steele, J., Fisher, J., McGuff, D., Bruce-Low, S., and Smith, D., "Resistance Training to Momentary Muscular Failure Improves Cardiovascular Fitness in Humans: A Review of Acute Physiological Responses and Chronic Physiological Adaptations." *Journal of Exercise Physiology On-Line*, 15 no. 3 (June 2012) 53–80.

4. Messier, S.P., and Dill, M.E., "Alterations in strength and maximum oxygen consumption consequent to nautilus circuit weight training." *Res Q Exerc Sport* 56 (1985) 345–51.

5. Koffler, K., Menkes, A., Redmond, A., et al., "Strength training accelerates gastrointestinal transit in middle-aged and older men." *Med Sci Sports Exerc* 24 (1992) 415–9.

6. Campbell, W., Crim, M., Young, C., et al., "Increased energy requirements and changes in body composition with resistance training in older adults." *Am J Clin Nutr* 60 (1994)167–75.

7. Hurley, B., "Does strength training improve health status?" *Strength Cond J* 16 (1994) 7–13.

8. Stone, M., Blessing, D., Byrd, R., et al., "Physiological effects of a short

term resistive training program on middle-aged untrained men." *Nat Strength Cond Assoc J* 4 (1982) 16–20.

9. Hurley, B., Hagberg, J., Goldberg A., et al. "Resistance training can reduce coronary risk factors without altering VO2 max or percent body fat." *Med Sci Sports Exerc* 20 (1988) 150–4.

10. Harris K.A., Holly R.G., "Physiological responses to circuit weight training in borderline hypertensive subjects." *Med Sci Sports Exerc* 19 (1987) 246–52.

11. Colliander, E.B., Tesch, P.A., "Blood pressure in resistance trained athletes." *Can J Appl Sport Sci* 13 (1988) 31–4.

12. Menkes A., Mazel S., Redmond A., et al., "Strength training increases regional bone mineral density and bone remodelling in middle-aged and older men." *J Appl Physiol* 74 (1993) 2478–84.

13. Rall, L.C., Meydani S.N., Kehayias, J.J., et al., "The effect of progressive resistance training in rheumatoid arthritis: increased strength without changes in energy balance or body composition." *Arthritis Rheum* 39 (1996) 415–26.

14. Nelson, B.W., O'Reilly E., Miller, M., et al., "The clinical effects of intensive specific exercise on chronic low back pain: a controlled study of 895 consecutive patients with 1-year follow up." *Orthopedics* 18 (1995) 971–81.

15. Risch, S., Nowell, N., Pollock, M., et al., "Lumbar strengthening in chronic low back pain patients." *Spine* 18 (1993) 232–8.

16. Westcott W., "Keeping Fit." *Nautilus* 4 (1995) 50–7.

17. Messier, S.P., Dill, M.E., "Alterations in strength and maximum oxygen consumption consequent to nautilus circuit weight training." *Res Q Exerc Sport* 56 (1985) 345–51.

18. Stone, M.H., "Muscle conditioning and muscle injuries." *Med Sci Sports Exerc* 22 (1990) 457–62.

19. Melov, Simon, et al., "Resistance Exercise Reverses Aging in Human Skeletal Muscle." Published online at: http://www.plosone.org/article/info:doi%2F10.1371%2Fjournal.pone.0000465

20. http://www.cbc.ca/news/health/weight-training-staves-off-dementia-in-older-women-1.1188553

CHAPTER THIRTEEN

1. According to Shellock and Prentice (1985), most of the physiological effects of warm up are temperature dependent. Muscle contraction requires the breaking of adenosine trip-phosphate (ATP) to provide the energy for cross-bridge formation (See "Sliding Element Mechanism," Norkin and Levangie, 2000, p. 277). According to Marieb (1998), only 20–25 percent of the energy produced through muscle contraction goes toward directly functional work. The remaining 75–80 percent is given off as heat. It is this heat that caused the rise in tissue temperature that is so advantageous to the athlete. The physiological effects of raised muscle temperature are numerous. Increased body temperature increases oxygen delivery to the working tissues by facilitating oxygen dissociation from hemoglobin and myoglobin (Shellock and Prentice, 1985). Vasodilation occurs as a result of increased temperature and waste production (Karvonen, 1978). Local vasodilation redistributes blood from the viscera to working muscles. This shunting of blood flow allows increased nutrient and oxygen delivery and improves the efficiency of waste product removal.

CHAPTER FOURTEEN

1. DeSimone, William., *Congruent Exercise: How To Make Weight Training Easier On Your Joints* (CreateSpace, 2011), 15.
2. Burd, Nicholas A., et al., "Influence of Muscle Contraction Intensity And Fatigue On Muscle Protein Synthesis (MPS) Following Resistance Exercise." *Medicine & Science in Sports & Exercise*, 41 no. 5 (May 2009), 149.

CHAPTER FIFTEEN

1. Clarkson, P.M., and Nosaka, K., "Muscle function after exercise-induced muscle damage and rapid adaptation." *Medicine and Science in Sports and Exercise* 24, No.5 (1992), 512–20.
2. Clarkson, P.M., and Tremblay, I., "Exercise-induced muscle damage, repair and adaptation in humans." *Journal of Applied Physiology* 65 no. 1 (1988), 1–6.
3. Friden, J., et al, "Myofibrillar damage following intense eccentric

exercise in man." *International Journal of Sports Medicine*, 24 no. 3 (1983), 170–176.

4. Golden, C.L., and Dudley, G.A., "Strength after bouts of eccentric or concentric actions." *Medicine and Science in Sports and Exercise*, 24 no. 8 (1992), 926–33.

5. Howell, J.N., Chleboun, G., "Muscle stiffness, strength loss, swelling and soreness following exercise-induced injury to humans." *Journal of Physiology* 464 (1993), 183–96.

6. Jones, D.A., Newham, J.M., et al, "Experimental human muscle damage: morphological changes in relation to other indices of damage." *Journal of Physiology* 375 (1986), 435–48.

7. Mishra, D.K., Friden, J., et al., "Anti-inflammatory medication after muscle injury." *Journal of Bone and Joint Surgery*, 77-A no.10 (1995), 1510–19.

8. Newman, D.J., Jones, D.A., "Repeated high-force eccentric exercise: effects on muscle pain and damage." *Journal of Applied Physiology* 4 no. 63 (1987), 1381–86.

9. Smith, L.L., "Acute inflammation: the underlying mechanism in delayed onset muscle soreness?" *Medicine and Science in Sports and Exercise* 23, no.5 (1991), 542–51.

10. Tiidus, P.M., and Ianuzzo, D.C.. "Effects of intensity and duration of muscular exercise on delayed soreness and serum enzyme activities." *Medicine and Science in Sports and Exercise*, 15, no.6 (1983) 461–5.

11. Graves et al., "Effect of reduced training frequency on muscular strength." *Int J Sports Med* 9 no. 5 (Oct. 1988), 316–9. PubMed #3246465. According to the researchers:

    > Strength values for subjects who reduced training to 2 and 1 days/week were not significantly different.... These data suggest that muscular strength can be maintained for up to 12 weeks with reduced training frequency.

12. Graves et al., "Effect of training frequency and specificity on isometric lumbar extension strength." *Spine* 15 no. 6 (1990), 504–9. PubMed #2144914. The researchers concluded:

    > These data indicate that a training frequency as low as 1X/week provides an effective training stimulus for the development of lumbar extension strength.

13. DeRenne., "Effects of Training Frequency on Strength Maintenance in Pubescent Baseball Players." *Journal of Strength and Conditioning Research* 10 (1996). The researchers concluded:

   . . . for pubescent male athletes, a 1-day-a-week maintenance program is sufficient to retain strength during the competitive season.

14. Taaffe et al., "Once-weekly resistance exercise improves muscle strength and neuromuscular performance in older adults." *J Am Geriatr Soc.* 47, no. 10 (1999), 1208–14. PubMed #10522954. The participants in the study were divided into three groups that trained once, twice or three days per week. All three groups became equally stronger, causing the researchers to conclude:

   A program of once or twice weekly resistance exercise achieves muscle strength gains similar to 3 days per week training in older adults.

15. McLester et al., "Comparison of 1 Day and 3 Days per Week of Equal-Volume Resistance Training in Experienced Subjects." *Journal of strength and conditioning research* (2000). The researchers concluded:

   The findings suggest that a higher frequency of resistance training, even when volume is held constant, produces superior gains in 1RM. However, training only 1 day per week was an effective means of increasing strength, even in experienced recreational weight trainers.

16. DiFrancisco-Donoghue et al., "Comparison of once-weekly and twice-weekly strength training in older adults." *British Journal of Sports Medicine* 41 no. 1 (2007), 19–22. PubMed #17062657. The researchers concluded that:

   One set of exercises performed once weekly to muscle fatigue improved strength as well as twice a week in the older adult. Our results provide information that will assist in designing strength-training programmes that are more time and cost efficient in producing health and fitness benefits for older adults.

17. Burt et al., "A comparison of once versus twice per week training on leg press strength in women." *J Sports Med Phys Fitness* 47 no.1 (2007), 13–17. PubMed #17369792. The researchers concluded that:

These results indicate that performing a single set of the leg press once or twice per week results in statistically similar strength gains in untrained women.

CHAPTER SEVENTEEN

1. http://digg.com/2016/calorie-unit-broken
2. http://www.webmd.com/diet/20090511/obesity-epidemic-overeating-alone-to-blame
3. Ibid.
4. https://newsnetwork.mayoclinic.org/discussion/are-you-getting-too-much-protein/

ABOUT THE AUTHOR

John Little is considered "one of the top fitness researchers in North America" (*Ironman* magazine). An accomplished author in the field of exercise (*Max Contraction Training, Body By Science, The Art of Expressing the Human Body*), philosophy, history, and martial arts, Little's articles have been published in every major fitness and martial arts magazine in North America. Throughout his career, Little has worked alongside the biggest names in the industry, from the Estate of Bruce Lee to bodybuilding icons such as Arnold Schwarzenegger, Mike Mentzer, Steve Reeves, and Lou Ferrigno to action stars such as Jackie Chan. Little is also an award-winning documentary filmmaker, having produced and directed films for both independent companies and major studios such as Warner Bros. Little and his wife, Terri, opened Nautilus North Strength & Fitness Centre in 2004, where they continue to conduct studies on exercise and share the data with their personal training clients. Nautilus North has supervised in excess of eighty thousand one-on-one workout sessions. Little lives in Bracebridge, Ontario (Canada), with Terri and their children Riley, Taylor, Brandon, and Benjamin.